Caring for Children with Special Healthcare Needs and Their Families

A Handbook for Healthcare Professionals

CARING FOR CHILDREN WITH SPECIAL HEALTHCARE NEEDS AND THEIR FAMILIES

A Handbook for Healthcare Professionals

Editor
Linda L. Eddy, PhD, RN, CPNP
Associate Professor
College of Nursing
Washington State University
Vancouver, Washington, USA

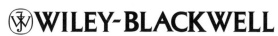
WILEY-BLACKWELL

A John Wiley & Sons, Inc., Publication

Editorial offices: 2121 State Avenue, Ames, Iowa 50014-8300, USA
The Atrium, Southern Gate, Chichester, West Sussex, PO19 8SQ, UK
9600 Garsington Road, Oxford, OX4 2DQ, UK

For details of our global editorial offices, for customer services and for information about how to apply for permission to reuse the copyright material in this book please see our website at www.wiley.com/wiley-blackwell.

Library of Congress Cataloging-in-Publication Data

Caring for children with special healthcare needs and their families : a handbook for healthcare professionals / editor, Linda L. Eddy, PhD, RN, CPNP, associate professor, College of Nursing, Washington State University Vancouver, Vancouver, Washington, USA.
    pages   cm
  Includes bibliographical references and index.
    ISBN 978-0-8138-2082-8 (pbk. : alk. paper) – ISBN (invalid) 978-1-118-51794-9 (emobi) – ISBN 978-1-118-51796-3 (epdf/ebook) – ISBN 978-1-118-51797-0 (epub)   1. Children with disabilities–Care.   2. Parents of children with disabilities   3. Child health services.
I. Eddy, Linda L., editor of compilation.
  RJ138.C43 2013
  362.4–dc23
                                                                                    2012039435

A catalogue record for this book is available from the British Library.

Cover design by Nicole Teut

Set in 10/12.5pt Sabon by Aptara® Inc., New Delhi, India
Printed and bound in Malaysia by Vivar Printing Sdn Bhd

1   2013

This book is dedicated to my son, Erik, without whom this book would not have come to be. Erik was born in 1980 with severe physical and developmental disabilities and it was through him that I learned the most important lessons about caring for children with disabilities, and about helping their parents take care of themselves and others in their lives. These lessons were learned, in part, through painful losses and hard fought personal and professional battles. Erik was the inspiration and catalyst for my 26-year academic and primary care practice career with children with disabilities and their families. My hope is that my healthcare colleagues and friends, as well as interested families and caregivers, will benefit from what I have learned, as well as from the contributions of my colleagues who have also benefitted from the children and families who have graced their lives.

CONTENTS

Sheela M. Choppala-Nestor, PhD,
PMHNP-BC, APRN
Clinical Director
Associates for Psychiatric and
Mental Health, LLC
Vancouver, Washington, USA

Phyllis Eide, PhD, MPH, MN,
APRN-BC
Associate Professor
College of Nursing
Washington State University
Spokane, Washington, USA

Linda L. Eddy
Associate Professor
College of Nursing
Washington State University
Vancouver, Washington, USA

Ginny Wacker Guido, JD, MSN,
RN, FAAN
Regional Director for Nursing and
Assistant Dean
College of Nursing
Washington State University
Vancouver
Vancouver, Washington, USA

Janet A. Lohan, Ph.D., RN, CPN
Clinical Associate Professor
College of Nursing
Washington State University
Spokane, Washington, USA

Nancy Lowry MN, RN
Public Health/Community
Consultant
Oregon Center for Children &
Youth with Special Health Needs
Oregon Health & Science University
Portland, Oregon, USA

Lisa Lyons, Ph.D., CCC-SLP
Legacy Health System

Portia Riley, MFT, LMHC
Family Therapist
Hospital Intake Coordinator
Community Services Northwest
Vancouver, Washington, USA

Jeannine Roth, RN, MSN, CPN
College of Nursing
Washington State University
Vancouver, Washington, USA

Patricia Shaw RN, BSN
Program Manager
Children with Special Health Care
Needs Program
Clark County Public Health
Vancouver, Washington, USA

Mary C. Sobralske, PhD, RN
Family Nurse Practitioner
Shriners Hospitals for Children-
Honolulu, Hawaii
Spokane, Washington USA

Caring for Children with Special Healthcare Needs and Their Families

A Handbook for Healthcare Professionals

CHAPTER 1
INTRODUCTION

Linda L. Eddy

Caring for Children with Special Healthcare Needs and Their Families: A Handbook for Healthcare Professionals, First Edition. Edited by Linda L. Eddy.

In 2010, data from the national *Survey of Children with Special Health Care Needs* indicated that approximately 15% of children in the United States had special healthcare needs. With a population this large, it is likely that most pediatric healthcare professionals will have occasion to care for this population of children and their families in a variety of outpatient and inpatient settings in the community. Many clinicians, however, have limited experience with meeting the needs of children with disabilities and may feel uncomfortable with their care. Clinicians can significantly influence overall health and well-being by offering interventions that influence the well-being, levels of support, and stress levels of both children with disabilities and their parents. Taking a family approach is important not only for the adults but also because of the link between child well-being and parent well-being. Thus, the goal of this handbook is to provide a resource that is easily accessible to clinicians from a variety of disciplines, and that offers concrete, practical suggestions for caring for children with physical, sensory, developmental, communication, and social/emotional challenges. This text is likely to be of benefit to professionals from the fields of nursing, social work, physical therapy, occupational therapy, and speech therapy, among others. Although the primary focus of the handbook is on caring for children with disabilities in the United States, the organizing frameworks and major concepts presented in each chapter have cross-cultural relevance. We hope that this handbook will meet the needs of clinicians in practice. For this reason, the chapters are presented in an expanded outline format so that key material can be easily accessed, and each chapter offers suggested interventions that are highlighted.

The handbook is organized into three main content areas:

- Chapters 2 and 3 examine common features of a variety of physical, sensory, and developmental disabilities. Descriptions include etiologies, presenting signs and symptoms, prognosis, common therapies, and an introduction to roles of healthcare providers that are often a part of interprofessional teams caring for children with disabilities.

- Chapters 4 through 6 shift the focus away from recognizing and understanding a particular disability and toward specific interventions addressing differences common to children with a variety of special needs, including differences in community, mobility, and social/emotional status.

- Chapters 7 through 13 broaden the scope to inform clinicians about cross-cutting issues affecting children with disabilities in a variety of settings. We address the role of the family as client, legal and regulatory issues, theoretical bases for quality care, enhancement of the child's and family's quality of life, the role of public health and school nursing professionals, end-of-life care, care planning, and coordination of care.

INTRODUCTION

We hope that by moving from a narrow focus on specifics to a broader perspective of the child and family in a variety of contexts that we are able to meet both immediate and longer-term needs of clinicians in practice. Throughout the handbook, the editor offers case examples from her practice as a pediatric nurse practitioner. One case in particular, from the editor's practice as a pediatric nurse practitioner with children with special needs, offers a number of promising practices for high-quality care of children with special needs and their families, as well as examples of challenges inherent in caring for this population. Exemplars of practice, such as this case, will be referenced throughout the remainder of the text.

- This is the story of Mia and her family. Mia is a five-year-old child with Down Syndrome who came into our outpatient pediatric clinic because of complaints of ear pain. Our staff was very familiar with Mia and very comfortable with her mother's knowledge about otitis media. I examined her, prescribed an antibiotic, and did the necessary teaching for safe administration. Although as pediatric primary care providers we often choose a "watch and wait" approach to treatment of otitis media in typically developing five-year-olds, children with Down Syndrome have some anatomical differences in the ear that put them at greater risk from complications related to otitis media.

  What I did less well was to inquire about the family system, and how they were adjusting to her diagnosis of Down Syndrome and all that entails. This memory stays with me many years later, as I have a child with severe disabilities and those early years were devastating to our family. Still, probably due to "being too busy," I did not take the time to make sure all was well. The next time I saw the family in the clinic all was clearly *not* well. Even though Mia presented with a similar complaint, her ears were fine but her family was not. This time her father was with Mia and her mother, and there was noticeable tension in the room. After assuring the family that Mia's ears were not infected, I asked "how is everything else going?" At this point, Mia's mother burst into tears, her father grabbed her, and they walked out of the examination room. Mia's mother told me that they had just received a letter from their local public school that outlined Mia's special education setting for her kindergarten year that fall. Apparently (and unsurprisingly) Mia's mother had been receiving lots of support from other parents of children with disabilities, but her father had been more or less denying the diagnosis and talking about her future as if the Down Syndrome did not exist. The letter from the school system eroded his denial and he was very angry. At this point in the encounter, one of my colleagues played with Mia in the waiting room and I spent time listening to Mia's parents talk and grieve, helping them make plans to move on. I was able to make some referrals for counseling and support that they requested, as well as help them develop a plan for respite care so that they might strengthen their ties as a couple. If I had only done this on the previous visit, this visit might have been unnecessary.

Although the first encounter demonstrates the importance of understanding growth and developmental differences in order to provide appropriate health promotion and disease prevention education for Mia, as well as the important role of the family as the context for high-level wellness in the child, the second encounter demonstrates a higher level of care with the entire family as the client.

INTRODUCTION

CHAPTER 2

COMMON PHYSICAL OR SENSORY DISABILITIES

Mary C. Sobralske

This chapter examines common features of physical and sensory disabilities often encountered in children and adolescents and discusses ways to foster quality of life for children and adolescents with these disabilities. These disorders often affect the lives of children and their families in profound ways; therefore they need healthcare and social services from specialists with a range of expertise.

CEREBRAL PALSY

Many healthcare providers misunderstand the term and etiology of cerebral palsy (CP) (Paneth, 2008). This is in part due to the fact that there are many aspects that even specialists do not understand about this disorder. It is important that healthcare providers have a clear understanding of what is commonly referred to as CP.

"Cerebral" means brain and "palsy" refers to a physical disorder that is characterized by a lack of muscle control. CP is not caused by problems with the muscles or nerves, but rather with the brain's ability to adequately control the body (www.cerebralpalsy.org). CP affects the central nervous system; it is a disorder of movement, coordination, muscle control, posture, and sometimes cognition. Depending on the cause of CP, when brain trauma likely occurred, and in what part of the brain, the effects of CP vary from individual to individual child.

Diagnosis, etiology, and risk factors of CP

Cerebral palsy is neither hereditary nor contagious. The etiology of CP is sometimes unclear; in up to 25–50% of cases of CP the cause is undetermined (www.cerebralpalsy.org, 2010). CP occurs in 2–4 out of every 1000 births in the United States. Certain risk factors are often present, and the cause can be explained by what most likely affected the brain. Based on national research, Nehring (2010) has listed over 40 risk factors for CP. Common risk factors for CP include maternal factors such as diabetes, infection, bleeding, and seizure disorders. Poor maternal health and maternal viral infections such as rubella, varicella, cytomegalovirus, toxoplasmosis, and syphilis can cause CP in the fetus.

Complications of labor and delivery are probably the ones best known by the lay public because they get the most notoriety. These include premature delivery at fewer than 37 weeks gestation, fetal heart rate depression, preeclampsia, abnormal fetal head presentation, prolonged rupture of membranes, long labor, and asphyxia (McGrath & Hardy, 2011).

COMMON PHYSICAL OR SENSORY DISABILITIES

Premature birth, low birth weight, breech presentation, intrauterine stroke, oxygen deprivation, and severe jaundice can cause CP (McGrath & Hardy, 2011; Mello et al., 2009). Perinatal risk factors include sepsis, seizures, intraventricular hemorrhage, meconium aspiration, low birth weight, and intrauterine growth retardation. Postnatal or infant brain insults that can cause CP include meningitis, viral encephalitis, traumatic brain injury, infection, and exposure to toxins. Congenital brain malformations and genetic syndromes can inhibit normal fetal brain development and can contribute to a diagnosis of CP.

Diagnosing CP usually involves extensive testing and imaging studies. Developmental and neurological tests are often the first step in making a diagnosis and finding the cause. Pediatric healthcare providers, teachers, and parents will often be the first to notice developmental problems (Harris, 2009). When making the diagnosis it is crucial to rule out other disorders that can cause movement problems similar to CP.

Developmental tests include many that are discussed elsewhere in this book. The Battelle Developmental Inventory (Newborg, 2004) is an assessment for infants and children through age 7. It is a flexible, semi-structured assessment that involves observation of the child, interviews with parents and caregivers, developmental and social history, and interaction with the child using game-like materials, toys, questionnaires, and tasks. The Denver Developmental Screening Test (Frankenburg & Dobbs, 1967) screens for cognitive and behavioral problems in preschool children.

Laboratory tests are mainly used to rule out conditions that may mimic CP or to determine why a fetus experienced a brain insult that caused CP. An example would be a blood-clotting disorder such as Factor V Leiden. Metabolic conditions such as phenylketonuria can prevent the brain from developing properly, causing symptoms similar to those of CP. Genetic tests can help determine if there are underlying genetic or congenital syndromes that account for the clinical presentation, rather than a brain insult. Testing is generally initiated by a genetic specialist.

Imaging studies commonly performed can help pinpoint the location of the underlying brain abnormality and sometimes provide the etiology (Paneth, 2008). These include computed tomography (CT), a sophisticated imaging technique that uses X-rays and a computer to create an anatomical picture of brain tissues and structures. A CT scan may reveal areas of the brain that are underdeveloped or have physical defects such as abnormal cysts. CT scans can also help determine the long-term prognosis of the child with CP.

Magnetic resonance imaging (MRI) is an imaging study that identifies many brain disorders. It uses magnetic fields and radio waves that produce pictures of structures and abnormal areas in the soft tissues of the head. A brain MRI will reveal stroke infarcts and masses.

If a child with CP has a seizure disorder, electroencephalogram (EEG) may be used in order to determine the cause of the seizures. EEG uses electrode patches placed on the scalp to record electrical activity suggesting seizures inside the brain.

Feeding studies in children with nutritional problems may be conducted under the supervision of a gastroenterologist or nutritional specialist to detect specific problems contributing to feeding difficulties. Genetic studies may be performed under the supervision of a geneticist in order to evaluate and diagnose conditions that have a familial disposition or are hereditary. Metabolic tests will often help diagnose the absence or insufficient amount of specific enzymes such as amino acids, vitamins, or carbohydrates necessary to maintain the normal chemical function of the body.

Presenting signs and symptoms of CP

Presenting signs and symptoms of CP are sometimes seen immediately after birth or even prenatally. More often, however, the diagnosis of CP is not made until the child starts developing as an infant or toddler and there are noticeable or detected delays in growth and development, and perhaps abnormal motor function. The effects of CP are categorized into one of four categories determined by the type of movement disorder, level of disability, lack of function, quality of life, and associated health problems and impairments. The four types include spasticity, dystonia, athetosis, and ataxia.

Spasticity

In a child with spastic CP the clinician notes increased muscle tone, persistent primitive reflexes, amplified stretch reflexes, a positive Babinski reflex, and ankle clonus (Nehring, 2010). Spastic CP is the most common type of movement disorder; it can involve all four extremities or just one. With spasticity there is motor dysfunction. Children may have tremors and periods of hypertonia and hypotonia between the spastic movements. Hypertonia is increased muscle tone or strength, and hypotonia is decreased muscle tone and strength.

Dystonia

Dystonia is impairment in muscle tone and movement in which sustained muscle contractions cause twisting and repetitive movements or abnormal postures.

Sometimes dystonia is painful and can affect the arms, legs, trunk, neck, eyelids, face, and vocal cords.

Athetosis

Athetosis is continual slow, flowing, writhing motions most often occurring in the hands and feet. These movements are involuntary, purposeless, and rigid. Athetoid movement is caused by disruption of the internal sensorimotor feedback system. Children with athetoid CP have difficulty holding themselves in the upright and steady positions required for them to sit and walk.

Ataxia

Ataxia is the inability to coordinate voluntary muscle movements. This produces uncoordinated movements and often a staggering gait, giving the appearance of clumsiness, imbalance, and instability. There is a concurrent lack of depth perception.

Classification of CP

It may be difficult to classify each child with CP because there are so many variables. Generally, CP is classified by the extremities involved, severity of neuromotor involvement, and ability to function. Hemiplegia is mainly manifested by lack of function or abnormal function in the arm and leg of one side; however, the entire side is affected in some way. "Hemi" means half or one-sided and "plegia" means paralysis. Children categorized as having hemiplegic CP generally have one side of their body affected by the brain insult when one of the hemispheres of the brain is damaged. Preference for one side of the body may present as asymmetric crawling and favoring one leg while climbing stairs. "Hemiparesis" is the term used when one half of the body is weakened but not paralyzed. "Monoplegia" is paralysis of one limb, usually an arm. This is the mildest form of cerebral palsy, and it heralds a good prognosis for the future. Early, abnormal hand preference in a child fewer than 3 years old is a sign of one-sided CP. Generally children do not have a hand preference until the age of 3. "Diplegia" is a form of CP in which both the arms and legs have abnormal stiffness or spasticity; however the legs are mostly affected by hypertonia and spasticity with little or no involvement of the arms. This form of CP is sometimes referred to as Little's disease (www.cerebralpalsy.org). "Quadriplegia" means that all four extremities are affected by the brain insult. This is the most severe type of CP, and children with quadriplegia will have the most complications.

Prognosis and complications

The prognosis of CP is not always predictable and will depend on the cause, severity, and type of CP (Nehring, 2010). Many factors affect the progression of problems and complications in CP. For example, some children develop neuromuscular scoliosis because of muscle imbalance and seating problems. Seating problems can lead to skin breakdown and pressure ulcers (Newman et al., 2010). Children with CP often have problems with learning, and feeding and eating problems are common, leading to nutritional impediments. If complications can be prevented, prognosis is excellent and some individuals with CP can live well into their 50s and 60s. If they develop complications such as skin ulcers and respiratory infections, or have other comorbidities, living into adulthood can be less likely (Jones, Morgan, & Shelton, 2007; Nehring). Parents should know that although children may develop progressive and chronic problems because of CP over time, the brain insult or abnormality causing CP does not progress or get worse; CP is a nonprogressive neurological deficit.

The ability to ambulate with their own legs or by use of a wheelchair increases childrens' independence. The ability to ambulate in the community and being independent are excellent predictors that longevity of life can be achieved. It is more likely that these individuals can also be productive citizens and less burdensome to the family and healthcare system. Being dependent on others to care for them and not being able to communicate puts many people with CP, usually severe, at risk for a multitude of problems. Life expectancy is related to the ability to take food by mouth and to any independent mobility the child has, including rolling and crawling. Children who are fully ambulatory and who self-feed have a life expectancy that is similar to children without a disability (Eyman, Grossman, Chaney, & Call, 1990).

Muscles of the pharynx and larynx may be spastic or hypotonic. This can cause the child to be prone to choking, aspiration, feeding problems, and speech disorders. Choking and aspiration may lead to gastroesophageal reflux, pneumonia, chronic bronchitis, and asthma (Nehring, 2010; Jones et al., 2007). Because of feeding problems, drooling, lack of motor control, and self-care deficits, children with CP may have more dental problems than average (Waldman, Perlman, & Rader, 2010). Side effects of medications such as anticonvulsants and muscle relaxants can also add to dental problems. Behavioral and emotional problems may make it difficult to maintain adequate oral hygiene.

Spasticity in CP causes a high caloric demand because the child is constantly moving, which requires a tremendous amount of energy expenditure. Thus, children with spasticity are often underweight, and undernutrition is common. Sometimes children cannot get enough calories to override the energy requirements of continual spastic movement. Facial and oral muscle tone may also be compromised, making it difficult for the child to eat many foods or drink. Excessive drooling, choking, and difficulty swallowing and sucking affect the intake of food. The inability to bring the hand to the mouth and hold a utensil and fingers to the mouth may be issues. It may take a caregiver or parent over an hour to feed a child a simple meal. Food may not always reach the mouth and be swallowed and digested. There may be much food wastage. Safety may also be an issue.

Common pharmacologic and non-pharmacologic therapies

CP is a life-long condition that is not correctable; therefore managing it means focusing on preventing or minimizing deformities and maximizing the child's capabilities at home and in the community. Therapies help children cope with their condition in the best way possible. Management of CP includes both non-surgical and surgical options. The literature discusses approaches to treatment and care based on the child's ability and function.

Many children with CP also have visual problems (Jones et al., 2007). Children may require glasses at a very early age. Contact lenses may be difficult to use for most children because they lack the fine motor dexterity and control required to insert and maintain contact lenses. Keeping glasses on the face in an orderly and clean fashion may be challenging. Nehring (2010) recommends securing glasses on to the face by using Velcro straps.

Physical and orthopedic manifestations of CP are treated by several specialists working together. Orthopedic care strives to improve placement and function of the tendons, bones, and joints, and to correct the position of the extremities that may have contractures. Nerves, muscles, and tendons may be severed (tenotomy) or lengthened to help reduce pain and contractures. Tight hip adductors such as the psoas major muscle can cause hip subluxation and dislocation over time.

CP is often treated by a rehabilitation team composed of physical therapy, occupational therapy, speech therapy, and audiology. Children with CP may need leg braces, special walkers, or a wheelchair. They may benefit from special orthotic shoes. Nonsurgical interventions may include rehabilitation; positioning aids to help children sit, lie, or stand; braces and splints used to prevent deformities and provide support or protection, and medications used to help control seizures or decrease spasticity in the muscles.

Orthotic devices for the arms and legs are used to provide stability to the joints, to help maintain joint range of motion, and to prevent or minimize contractures. Splints, ankle-foot orthotics, and special shoes, as well as adaptive equipment such as special eating utensils and standing devices are made by orthotists or therapists (Nehring, 2010). Scooters, tricycles, and motorized and customized wheelchairs all serve the needs of many children by increasing their ability to participate in a variety of play and recreational activities.

Physical therapy encourages children to become as strong as possible so their gait and voluntary movements are improved. Stretching exercises help prevent or reduce the severity of contractures and deformities. Physical therapists can help exercise the muscles and gain better motion. Medications can lessen muscle spasticity. Surgery and mobile technology such as wheelchairs all benefit the child with CP. However, the idea that life-long therapy is crucial to maintain muscle tone, bone structure, and prevent dislocation of the joints is still being debated by researchers. The benefit versus cost of providing ongoing services is being questioned by schools and insurance companies. How long should therapy be provided, and if so how often and how much will it cost?

Hyperbaric oxygen therapy uses pressurized oxygen that is inhaled inside a hyperbaric chamber. It has been used to treat CP under the premise that improving oxygen availability to damaged brain cells can reactivate some of them to function normally. Its use in the treatment of CP is still controversial (O'Shea, 2008).

Pharmacologic therapy is often overseen by the primary care provider but many medications may be prescribed by specialists such as neurologists, orthopedic surgeons, and gastroenterologists. Orthopedic problems may include scoliosis of the spine, hip dislocations, ankle and foot deformities, and contracted muscles and tendons. Orthopedic surgeons may use injectable Botulinum Toxin A (Botox®). Injections of Botox directly into spastic muscles can help relieve muscle spasms and contractures, at least temporarily.

Seizures and neurological problems are quite common in CP. A neurologist (a physician who specializes in conditions of the brain, spinal cord, and nerves) and sometimes a neurosurgeon (a surgeon who specializes in operating on the brain and spinal cord) will be involved in the child's treatment. Pediatric pulmonologists might be involved if the child's respiratory capacity is impacted.

Before contractures fully develop, neurologists will often prescribe muscle relaxants such as diazepam (Valium®), dantrolene (Dantrium®), and baclofen (Lioresal®). Oral baclofen causes many intolerable side effects and cannot be regulated continuously in the way that intrathecal (the subarachnoid space around the spinal cord) delivery of this drug can be. An intrathecal baclofen pump may be inserted for continual release of the medication in low doses. Older pumps are about the size of a small tuna can. Newer pumps are even smaller.

COMMON PHYSICAL OR SENSORY DISABILITIES

Botulinum toxin (Botox®), a highly effective treatment, is injected directly into the affected muscles by a neurologist or orthopedic specialist. Alcohol or phenol injections into the nerve controlling the muscle are other options. Multiple medications are available to control seizures, and athetosis can be treated using medications such as trihexyphenidyl HCl (Artane®) and benztropine (Cogentin®).

A gait analysis to evaluate the walking pattern of children may be performed in order to determine which therapies and orthotics may help.

Role of nursing

The role of nurses is critical in fostering quality of life for children and adolescents with CP. Nurses need to know that there are often comorbid health problems in children with CP. For these health-related problems, nurses are often in a good position to coordinate and monitor specialist interventions and interventions by other healthcare team members to assure that the child and the family are receiving all possible services to benefit the child. The goals of treatment for children with CP are to maintain mobility and ambulation, maximize range of motion of the joints, monitor muscle control and balance, enhance communication, receive adequate nutrition, and perform activities of daily living (World Health Organization, 2001). These goals will require comprehensive, multidisciplinary care across the child's life span (Nehring, 2010).

Nurses can perform a global assessment of the quality of life of the child and his or her family. This should include an assessment of the primary caregivers of children with CP.

For example, a mother of a teenage boy with CP was getting too old to lift her adolescent son from the wheelchair to his bed. No one else lived with them to help her in the household. She was afraid she would drop him or injure her son or herself in transferring him from the bed to a chair. She was already suffering chronic low back pain. The child weighed almost the same as his mother, and she needed services to help her manage her son's care.

The primary care needs of children with CP are similar to those of all children. For example, children should be able to receive all regularly scheduled childhood immunizations as recommended by the American Academy of Pediatrics (2011) with some exceptions. However, because children with seizure disorders are at increased risk of having a seizure after receiving pertussis vaccine, they should be given the acellular form of the vaccine along with tetanus and diphtheria (Broder et al., 2006). Hepatitis A vaccine should be given only if the child resides in an area with a high incidence of hepatitis

A and community prophylaxis is being conducted (Fiore, Wasley, Bell, 2006; Nehring, 2010).

Bowel and bladder function and toileting are major concerns for many children with CP. Because of low muscle tone or spastic abdominal muscles, constipation is common and often chronic (Nehring, 2010). Ways to treat and prevent constipation include exercise and adequate fluid intake. A high fiber diet, osmotic laxative medications that cleanse the bowel such as polyethylene glycol (MiraLAX®), proper positioning on the toilet or potty chair, and provision of a developmentally appropriate behavioral program may contribute to reducing the severity of bowel and bladder issues (American Academy for Cerebral Palsy and Developmental Medicine, 2011).

Nurses should assess whether children need a referral to a gastroenterologist or nutrition specialist if feeding and nutrition are problematic. A child may have severe enough problems with feeding that a gastrostomy tube, commonly called a G tube, or a jejunostomy tube, commonly called a J tube, are necessary. These tubes are surgically inserted into the stomach through the abdominal wall or into the jejunum, the small intestine. Although the child with a feeding tube receives most of their calories via the tube, some parents still feed their children a small amount of food orally, not so much for nutrition, but because the child enjoys the oral stimulation.

Nurses need to remember and remind parents and others that feeding skills develop sequentially (Jones et al., 2007). Children who are developmentally delayed are expected to eat based on their developmental age level, not based on their chronological age. A four-year-old girl might only be able to bottle-feed.

Roles of occupational and physical therapy

When a child with CP is very young, he or she will benefit greatly from physical therapy. Physical therapy can improve the development of milestones in motor function. Infants will often need assistance in learning to sit, crawl, stand up, and walk. Some children with CP will never walk, but that does not mean they cannot learn to ambulate using some form of equipment. Physical therapy prevents muscle weakness and deterioration. It can diminish muscle and tendon contractures. The goal is to make the child as functional as possible.

Occupational therapy will benefit children with upper extremity involvement. A child with CP may need special devices to learn to eat with utensils and/or chopsticks. As the child approaches preschool and grade school, special computers and learning devices may assist with communication and writing.

A child with CP may have difficulty with precise motions, such as writing or buttoning his shirt; excessive drooling; and difficulty swallowing, sucking, or speaking. There may be a lack of muscle coordination when performing voluntary movements, stiff muscles and exaggerated reflexes in spasticity, an asymmetrical walking gait, foot or leg dragging, and variations in muscle tone from too stiff to too floppy. All of these disruptions in normal movement can impair function. Using adaptive equipment may help with independence at school and in the community and with activities of daily living. Occupational therapists and OT assistants can determine the need for and create splints for the hands to help correct or prevent finger and wrist contractures. Children with CP often have difficulty doing more than one task at a time. OTs can teach children how to care for themselves and help them establish a sense of independence by doing simple tasks such as using the restroom by oneself or pulling one's shirt over one's head without help.

PTs and OTs will often perform tests on function. Some commonly used tests are the Bayley Motor Scale, the Peabody Developmental Motor Scale, the Alberta Infant Motor Scale, Children's Global Assessment Scale, Gross Motor Function Measure, and the Pediatric Evaluation of Disability Inventory.

Roles of speech and language therapy

Studies have shown that communication is one of the most problematic issues for children with CP (Russman, 2004). Speech impairments are commonly seen in CP, especially in those with oromotor deficits (Odding, 2006). Therefore, speech therapists play a vital part in treating some children with CP. Children with CP also may need testing for audiology. They may experience hearing deficits due to sensorineural damage or conductive hearing loss. Hearing deficits add to speech and communication problems. If they have a hearing impairment, they may need hearing aids. Speech therapists find ways to assist the child and family in communicating using sign language, adaptive devices, and alternative strategies such as use of pictures for doing schoolwork. Communication boards, switches, and sign language may be helpful. A speech therapist who specializes in augmentative communication is the most appropriate for a child who is nonverbal or has difficulty speaking (Jones et al., 2007). Some school systems have their own speech therapy program, which is a tremendous resource for children with CP.

A speech therapist can also help children strengthen their facial muscles if they are having trouble eating or swallowing, thus improving overall food intake and nourishment, and decreasing the risk of choking and aspiration. Speech specialists teach children how to carry on a conversation and give appropriate nonverbal cues such as eye contact. They also teach children

how to make important facial expressions and speak more clearly (www.cere
bralpalsy.org).

Roles of social work and psychology

Nurses should work closely together with social workers in coordinating care.
Safety and childcare, schooling and education, and dealing with cognitive disabilities and impairment in learning will all need to be addressed. Many cities
have support groups that can be located through the United Cerebral Palsy
Association, and most large medical centers have special multidisciplinary clinics for children with developmental disorders. Families who avail themselves
of CP support groups, family support services, patient advocacy programs, and
alternative educational services will benefit greatly. The United Cerebral Palsy
Association (http://www.ucpa.org) is one of the best resources for families.
Safety at home and in the community is highly important to address. Abuse of
children with developmental delays is a concern. Children are often vulnerable
to emotional, physical, and sexual abuse. Up to 60% of children with CP have a
cognitive impairment (United Cerebral Palsy Association) presenting a whole
host of problems. Children who are mentally retarded are especially vulnerable
to exploitation and abuse.

Positive reinforcement will encourage children to strengthen their self-esteem
and promote as much independence as possible. Advocating for ways the family can cope and get the support they need from community services will benefit
the family in the long term. The child's independence should be encouraged. A
supportive network can assist the family cope with CP and its effects. Parents
may feel grief and guilt over the child's disability. Social workers can find support groups, organizations, and counseling services in the child's community.
The child may benefit from family support programs, school programs, and
counseling.

Parents will want to know if subsequent children will be born with CP. It
is difficult to answer this question, as that will depend on the factors leading
to the CP and whether those factors can be eliminated in future childbearing
experiences.

Transition to adulthood

Transition occurs throughout the life span for every individual but particularly
difficult is the transition from adolescent to adult, especially for those with
special needs in general and CP in particular. Transitioning children from
pediatric to adult services is an ongoing challenge. Children may go from

pediatric primary care to less-coordinated care by a variety of adult healthcare providers. Adults will aim for autonomy: a goal not always realistic for adults with CP depending on the severity of symptoms.

Because individuals with CP often require services from several different types of healthcare professionals, transition to adult services can be particularly difficult. If children are receiving physical and occupational therapy, they may still require those services in adulthood. They will need a primary care provider who is experienced and/or trained in neuromotor disorders in adults. Educational needs and services will change. If the young adult attends college or vocational training, negotiation across campus from one building to the next can be a major barrier to getting an education. Weather can be an obstacle affecting ambulation in regions of the country that receives a heavy snow load or downpours. Elements such as below- freezing temperatures can be life-threatening. A student who ambulates by wheelchair or walker will need ample time to get from class to class. College professors may not have the training or experience working with students who have difficulty walking or who lack the motor skills to light up a Bunsen burner in chemistry lab. Modifications will need to be made, so the student and parents need to advocate for themselves with the help of the healthcare team.

The overall goal of transition care is to provide comprehensive, well-coordinated health, education, and vocational services (Sawin, Cox, & Metzger, 2010). Adults with CP, like most adults, want to be valued by society. They strive to develop meaningful relationships with other people and seek a sense of self-worth. They plan for the promise of a hopeful future and a successful life.

As for any young adult experiencing independent living, family planning and prevention of sexually transmitted infections are important issues (Wiegerink et al., 2006). Skills that young adults need to become independent in include domestic sills and personal hygiene. They need to know how to be safe, manage their finances, purchase necessary items from stores and the Internet, and find recreational and leisure activities they enjoy and can realistically do (Sawin et al., 2010).

Title V is legislation enacted by Congress in 1935 that specifically addresses health promotion and improvement for mothers and children in the United States. Title V originated in 1935 from the Maternal and Child Health Bureau as part of the Health Resources and Services Administration (US Department of Health and Human Services, 2011). Although certain laws exist, in reality not every community has the services necessary for the special needs of adults with CP. Often the focus of care for children with special health needs is to provide tertiary care. As more providers limit the number of patients insured by Medicaid, or at times even refuse to see these patients in their practice, emergency departments in hospitals are fast becoming where those with special health needs access their care. Barriers that exist are the lack of healthcare providers and their availability, proximity, and lack of comfort with diagnosing and treating CP.

In severe CP, an adult group home may be the most appropriate solution to caring for the adult person with CP, especially if the family can no longer provide the care the individual needs. It is important to find a group home whose mission and staff philosophy and experience is conducive to the needs of the individual with CP.

NEURAL TUBE DEFECTS (MYELODYSPLASIA/SPINA BIFIDA)

Spina bifida is a general term used to describe defects in the closure of the neural tube associated with malformations of the spinal cord and vertebra, called neural tube defect (NTD) (McGrath & Hardy, 2011; Spina Bifida Association, 2012). Included in this term are meningocele, or a presence of a sac containing meninges and cerebrospinal fluid; and myelomeningocele, or a presence of a sac containing meninges, cerebrospinal fluid, spinal cord, and nerve roots. Neural tube closure begins in the third to fourth week of gestation. An NTD, which can occur at any level of the spinal cord, occur in 1 in 1500 births in the United States (Spina Bifida Association).

Myelomeningocele may be closed or open. Other forms of NTDs include a tethered spinal cord and an Arnold-Chiari malformation, which is a caudal displacement of the cerebellar tonsils and brainstem below the foramen magnus. This malformation is present in 80–85% of cases of open myelomeningocele.

Hydrocephalus can also be associated with NTDs. Infants with hydrocephalus will have an accumulation of fluid in their brain. The head will appear large and dysmorphic.

Since 1992, women of childbearing age have been advised to consume 0.4mg of folic acid daily to prevent NTDs in their children. The rate of NTDs has decreased 26% with an increase in folic acid consumption (CDC, 2008).

Etiology

The cause of NTD is not known, but a combination of genetic and environmental factors has been suspected. No single gene has been identified to cause it, but scientists do know it is autosomal recessive. Risk factors include metabolic conditions such as diabetes and phenylketonuria; maternal infections such as cytomegalovirus and rubella; exposure to teratogens such as anticonvulsant drugs; obesity; hyperthermia; and nutritional deficiencies, particularly folate deficiency (Mayo Clinic, 2011). A family history of NTD and being Caucasian or Hispanic increases risks.

Presenting signs and symptoms

If a woman is receiving thorough prenatal care, ultrasonic visualization of a neural tubal defect may be apparent in utero (Cameron & Moran, 2009). If there is a family history of spina bifida, a hydrocephalic fetus, or elevated maternal serum alpha-fetoprotein levels, an amniocentesis will often be performed (Hochberg, 2009).

The symptoms of neural tube defects vary from child to child depending on the type of defect. Children with spina bifida occulta may have no outward signs of this disorder. Closed neural tube defects are often recognized early in life due to an abnormal tuft or clump of hair or a small dimple or birthmark on the skin at the site of the spinal malformation (National Institute of Neurological Disorders and Stroke, 2012).

Meningocele and myelomeningocele generally involve a fluid-filled sac visible on the back protruding from the spinal cord. In meningocele, the sac may be covered by a thin layer of skin, whereas in most cases of myelomeningocele, there is no layer of skin covering the sac and a section of spinal cord tissue usually is exposed.

Depending on the size and location of the NTD, whether skin covers the lesion, and which spinal nerves are affected, neurological deficits vary from mild to severe. Neurological deficits are classified by the lowest functional motor levels:

- Thoracic - no lower extremity motor function

- L1-2 – hip flexors, hip adductors function

- L3-4 – quadriceps function

- L4-5 – hamstrings, dorsiflexors function

- Sacral – plantar flexors function.

Sensory deficits are not as profound as motor deficits. If sacral nerves are affected, there is loss of normal bowel and bladder function. The level of involvement will initially be assessed by ultrasonography, CT scan, or MRI scan.

At birth, physical findings indicating a NTD may include: an obvious spinal lesion, a large head circumference if hydrocephalus is associated with the NTD, a lack of spontaneous movement of the lower extremities, hip clicks secondary to developmental hip dysplasia, clubfoot, scoliosis, flaccid or spastic muscles in the legs, and abnormal urine and stool leakage (McGrath & Hardy, 2011).

Prognosis

Children with a NTD can lead relatively active lives. Prognosis depends on the number and severity of abnormalities and associated complications. Most children have normal intelligence and can walk, usually with assistive devices. If learning problems develop, early education is beneficial (National Institutes of Neurological Disorders and Stroke, 2010).

Associated problems include urinary tract infections, urinary reflux, incontinence, and toileting issues. Urinary tract infection (UTI) is the most frequently reported cause of mortality in adults with NTD. There may be a lack of sensation and therefore safety issues such as being unaware of burns. Maintaining skin integrity and preventing skin ulcers are challenges. Some children with NTDs are highly allergic to latex and similar rubber products and certain foods, such as bananas.

Having associated hydrocephalus, a seizure disorder, and cognitive deficits complicate NTDs. Seizures occur in up to 25% of children with NTDs because of related cerebral anomalies, central nervous system infections, multiple shunt failures, and a history of respiratory problems (Lazzaretti & Pearson, 2010). If children have a seizure disorder, they will probably be taking anticonvulsant medications, which have many side effects and long-term adverse problems. Cognitive delays can affect the prognosis of children with NTDs. Cognitive deficits may result from the NTD itself; however, the toll of brain insults over time can inhibit the development of cognitive skills.

Common pharmacologic and non-pharmacologic therapies

There is no known cure for nerve damage due to NTDs. The nerve tissue that is damaged or lost cannot be repaired or replaced, nor can function be restored to the damaged nerves (National Institute of Neurological Disorders, 2012). Meningocele requires neurosurgery to correct the malformed meninges and close the opening in the vertebrae. Myelomeningocele also requires surgery within several hours to several days after birth. Performing the surgery early can help minimize the risk of infection that is associated with exposed nerves and may also help protect the spinal cord from additional trauma. Closure

COMMON PHYSICAL OR SENSORY DISABILITIES

of the dural defect often results in changes of the cerebral spinal fluid that results in insufficient drainage, thus causing hydrocephalus (National institute of Neurological Disorders). A ventricular–peritoneal shunt may be surgically placed to provide a continuous drain for the cerebrospinal fluid. Shunts most commonly drain into the abdomen.

Children with a tethered spinal cord that is bound to the scar of the closure will be less able to properly grow in length (National Institute of Neurological Disorders, 2012). Progressive tethering can cause loss of muscle function to the legs, bowel, and bladder. Surgery can limit the degree of disability and may also restore some function.

Most children with NTDs need periodic evaluations by specialists such as orthopedists, neurosurgeons, and urologists. Care should begin immediately after birth. Ambulation and mobility are major concerns. Ambulation may require bracing and a scooter or wheelchair with special seating.

Most children need to see an orthotist for braces, crutches, walkers, or wheelchairs to maximize mobility. Generally, the higher the level of the NTD, the more severe the paralysis, but paralysis does not always occur. Thus, with low levels of involvement, only short leg braces are necessary and some children may be able to walk unaided. Children with higher-level involvement usually do best with a wheelchair.

The urinary system should be evaluated for infection, obstruction, reflux, and dysgenesis. For example, at the Child Development and Rehabilitation Center in Portland, Oregon, once the urinary system is evaluated, plans are made to prevent infection and damage due to ureteral reflux. The infant may require intermittent catheterization, prophylactic antibiotics, release of an obstruction, ureteral reimplantation, or cystostomy. Some children need to manage the urinary system with a program of catheterization. Medications used for urinary incontinence include anticholinergics such as Ditropen® and Detrol®. Antibiotics to treat urinary tract infections include amoxicillin, TMP-SMX such as Septra®, and nitrofurantoin (Lazzaretti & Pearson, 2010).

Most children require a bowel management program, though some may have normal function. Bowel management should focus on maintaining soft, formed stools with a schedule of regular defecation on the toilet every one to two days (Lazzaretti & Pearson, 2010). Assistive devices for proper toilet seating may be necessary. Medications often used are bulking agents, MiraLAX®, stool stimulants, stool softeners, and lubricants (Lazzaretti & Pearson).

The best way to treat a NTD is to prevent it in the first place. Therefore, folic acid as a supplement is taken at least one month before conception and during the first trimester of pregnancy to reduce the risk of NTDs when at all possible.

Folic acid dosage should be 400 μ g per day for women of childbearing age and 600–800 μ g per day if a woman already has one child with a NTD. Foods high in folic acid include beans, citrus fruits, egg yolks, and dark green vegetables. The dosage should not exceed 1 mg per day. Taking folic acid can reduce the incidence of NTD by 50% (US Preventive Task Force, 2009).

Roles of nursing

The Spina Bifida Association of America (2012) recommends certain standards of care. These standards aim to help children negotiate developmental stages, reach and maintain independence, and prevent known medical complications. Nurses are often in the best position to coordinate, monitor, and oversee specialist interventions to assure the child is receiving all possible services. The goals of treatment for children with NTDs are to maintain mobility and ambulation, perform activities of daily living, and reduce the incidence of urinary and bowel problems.

Nurses will likely be assisting primary care providers and families in monitoring and coordinating appointments with and care by specialists such as urologists, neurologists, orthopedic specialists, physical and occupational therapists, and nutritionists. In the larger cities of the United States, special programs may be available to children with NTDs making it much easier for families to negotiate the healthcare system.

The majority of nursing care will involve toileting issues. Bowel and bladder management is essential for the child with a NTD. Nurses need to be aware that children with NTDs often are allergic to rubber (latex) products. In Table 2.1, items commonly found in healthcare facilities that may contain rubber products are cited by the New York State Department of Health (2012) and the Spina Bifida Association (2012) potentially causing harm to children with latex allergies. Nutritional problems include allergies, sometimes severe, to latex-related foods, including bananas, avocados, gum, chestnuts, kiwis, and pears. Other allergens, such as poinsettias and milkweed, if ingested are potentially deadly. It is extremely important that parents, neighbors, friends, and teachers are aware of these sometimes life-threatening allergies.

Occupational and physical therapy

A physical therapist will evaluate movement range and quality and prescribe home therapies and stretching exercises to be done by the child with the assistance of the parents. Physical therapists will assist other professionals in planning for surgeries, orthotic braces, casting, and ambulation. Physical therapy

COMMON PHYSICAL OR SENSORY DISABILITIES

Table 2.1 Common Latex Products

• Medical and dental devices and equipment	• Ear plugs
• Balloons and balls	• Gloves
• Clothes with rubber elastic	• Enemas
• Condoms and diaphragms	• Respiratory and IV equipment
• Costumes	• Infection control equipment
• Sneakers and swimsuits	• Ostomy supplies
• Water toys and swimming equipment	• Medical vial stoppers
• Diapers and rubber pants	• Penrose drains
• Food handled with latex gloves	• Pulse oximeters
• Mattress pads	• Thermometer probes
• Newsprint	• Skin adhesives
• Pacifiers and feeding nipples	• Stethoscopes
• Paints and stains	• Suction tubing
• Rubber bands and erasers	• Tapes
• Bungee cords	• Disposable covers
• Toothbrushes with rubber grips	• Tourniquets
• Toys	• Therabands for therapy
• Band-Aids	• Tubing and sheeting
• Blood pressure cuffs and tubing	• Vascular and compression stockings
• Catheters	• Wheelchair cushions and tires
• Dressings	• Zippered plastic storage bags

Sources: New York State Department of Health. Latex Allergy Information for Health Professionals. May 2012. http://www.health.ny.gov/publications/1453/; www.spinabifidaassociation.org

can improve the development of milestones in motor function, enhance gross motor skills, and provide passive range of motion exercises.

School-based physical therapy (Tecklin, 2008) may include engaging in gait training, participating in a strengthening program for the trunk and arms, dealing with leg length discrepancy due to knee flexion contractures, conducting manual muscle testing, providing a shoe lift and orthotics, and offering swimming exercises and pool therapy when available.

Infants may need assistance in learning to sit, crawl, stand up, and walk. Some children with NTDs will never walk, but that does not mean they cannot learn to ambulate using some form of equipment. The goal is to make the child as functional as possible.

Speech and language therapy

Children with NTDs may have learning disabilities, attention problems, and visual deficits, and may miss days of school because of related health problems. Those children with concomitant hydrocephalus may be hypersensitive to loud noises (Lazzaretti & Pearson, 2010). Therefore, some children may benefit from speech therapy. If nurses and parents have concerns about hearing and speech development, screening is recommended.

Social work and psychology

Having an infant born with a NTD can be devastating for parents. Many women are not even aware of their pregnancy until the mid- to later part of the first trimester. Grief, guilt, anger, fear, and sadness are emotional responses to hearing the news that their newborn has spina bifida. Therefore, it is important that families receive the support and knowledge that they need to make informed decisions and cope with what is in store. There are several support groups for families with a child with a NTD listed in the references at the end of this chapter. A social worker can review family health insurance, resources, and services, assess how well the family is coping, and determine community and home support needs.

As with any children with disabilities, socialization with other children about the same age is important. Some children will have the opportunity to associate with other special needs children. The severity of the NTD will determine, in part, what types of activities the child will engage in. Some children will do what is typical for any child of that particular age, may keep up very well with their peers, and be easily integrated into their peer group. Others will not. Urinary and fecal management is imperative in social settings if children are going to be well accepted by nondisabled peers. It is important that families treat their children as regular family members and not focus all the attention on the child with NTDs (Lazzaretti & Pearson, 2010).

Transition to adulthood

The primary healthcare needs, independent living skills, vocational training, and socialization should be addressed in planning transition into adulthood (Lazzaretti & Pearson, 2010). In order for someone to live independently, a strong social support system is necessary. An independent adult must have the level of function and cognition to be able to live independently. This will vary from individual to individual. Helpful organizations are listed at the end of this chapter.

MUSCULAR DYSTROPHY

In addition to CP, other fairly common neuromuscular disorders include the muscular dystrophies. These disorders have effects on children and families that may be similar to those of CP. Many services that benefit children with CP will also benefit children with other neuromuscular disorders such as muscular dystrophy.

Muscular dystrophy (MD) is a group of inherited muscle diseases in which muscle fibers are unusually susceptible to damage (Mayo Clinic, 2011). Muscles become progressively weaker and in the late stages, fat and connective tissue often replace muscle fibers. Cardiac and other organ muscles sometimes are affected. The most common type of MD, called dystrophinopathy, is due to a genetic deficiency of the muscle protein dystrophin. Other more common types of MD include Duchennne's MD, Becker's MD, Myotonic dystrophy (also known as Steinert's disease), congenital myotonic dystrophy, and facioscapulohumeral MD.

Etiologies of muscular dystrophy

Each form of MD is caused by a genetic mutation particular to the type of disease. The disease can be an X-linked recessive inheritance pattern with the mother being the carrier, or may have an autosomal dominant inheritance pattern. Duchenne's MD, seen mostly in boys, is the most common and the most severe form of MD that affects children. It is passed from mother to son through one of the mother's genes. Boys inherit the X chromosome from mother and a Y chromosome from their father. The defective gene is located on the X chromosome. The disease can skip a generation until another son inherits the defective gene on the X chromosome. The disorder can also arise from a new gene mutation rather than from an inherited defective gene.

Presenting signs and symptoms

Signs and symptoms vary according to the type of muscular dystrophy. Presentation may include muscle weakness, lack of coordination, progressive crippling, muscle and tendon contractures, and loss of mobility. Duchenne's MD usually presents by the age of 3 to 6 years. The child may experience frequent falls; demonstrate a clumsy gait; develop large calf muscles (called pseudohypertrophy); or have difficulty climbing stairs, getting up from a reclined or sitting position, or arising from the floor (a positive neurological sign called the Gower test). Other signs and symptoms include weakness in the foreleg muscles, difficulty running and jumping, development of a waddling gait, and sometimes experiencing cognitive deficits and cardiac problems. Signs and symptoms usually appear by the age of 3. The disease first affects the muscles of the pelvis, upper arms, and upper legs. By late childhood, most children are unable to walk. Some children later develop scoliosis. Most children die in their late 20s and 30s due to complications such as respiratory muscle weakness, pneumonia, and cardiac complications.

Becker's MD, a milder form of dystrophinopathy, generally affects older boys and young men and progresses slowly over several decades (Mayo Clinic, 2011). Onset occurs about age 6 to 11. Children are usually able to walk well into adulthood. Symptoms are similar to Duchenne's MD but milder. The child may have myoglobinuria or discolored urine due to the muscle enzyme myoglobin breakdown in the kidneys. Muscle cramps are common, and the child may present with cardiomyopathy. There may be decreased proximal reflexes, sinus tachycardia, heel cord tightness, ocular abnormalities, toe walking, or swaying.

In myotonic dystrophy, there is stiffness of muscles and weakness of and an inability to relax muscles voluntarily, usually referred to as myotonia. Progression is slow and often does not affect a child's function until he or she is an adult. Most signs and symptoms will present later in adulthood. In congenital myotonic dystrophy, infants are affected and may have severe muscle weakness, hypotonia, difficulty sucking and swallowing, difficulty breathing, or cognitive impairment.

Diagnostic tests may include assessing levels of muscle enzymes such as serum creatine kinase (CK). Elevated levels of CK suggest muscle disease. Electromyography may be employed to confirm muscle disease by detecting changes in the pattern of electrical activity of the muscles. Ultrasound can detect muscle abnormalities in the early stages of the disease. Muscle biopsy and laboratory analysis can distinguish the specific type of muscular dystrophy and identify dystrophin and other biologic markers. Genetic testing can identify deletions or duplication on the dystrophin gene in about 65% of cases of MD. The child may need cardiac studies and pulmonary function tests to determine respiratory and cardiovascular status.

Prognosis

There is no known cure for muscular dystrophy. Inactivity, such as bed rest, and even sitting for long periods, can worsen the disease. Current treatment is targeted to help prevent or reduce deformities in the joints, muscles, and spine and to allow children with MD to remain mobile as long as possible. Genetic research holds promise for developing methodologies to halt the progression of the disease.

Common pharmacologic and non-pharmacologic therapies

Medications can slow the progression of MD and manage some of the symptoms. Myotonia, muscle spasms, stiffness, and weakness associated with MD are treated with the antiarrhythmic drug mexiletine (Mexitil®);

the anticonvulsant drugs phenytoin (Dilantin®, Phenytek®) and carbamazepine (Tegretol®, Carbatrol®), a derivative of gamma-aminobutyric acid called baclofen (Lioresal®) primarily used to treat spasticity; and dentrolene (Dantrium), a muscle relaxant that acts by abolishing excitation-contraction coupling in muscle cells. The anti-inflammatory corticosteroid prednisone may improve muscle strength and delay the progression of Duchenne's MD.

Immunosuppressive drugs such as cyclosporine (Sandimmune®) and azathioprine (Azasan®, Imuran®) may delay damage to dying muscle cells (Myoclinic.com). Cardiac problems that occur with some kinds of muscular dystrophies, particularly myotonic muscular dystrophy, may require a pacemaker. Myotonia, or delayed relaxation of a muscle after a strong contraction, occurring in myotonic muscular dystrophy, may be treated with medications such as quinine, phenytoin, or mexiletine, but no long-term treatment is available.

Stem cell research shows promise. Steroids may prolong the ability to walk and result in slower decline in physical function (King et al., 2007). Respiratory therapy such as incentive spirometry and positive pressure ventilation may be necessary as the disease progresses.

Roles of nursing

As in other neuromuscular diseases, children will need comprehensive primary care and monitoring and coordination of specialized care. Children with MD are at high risk for medical complications. Nurses will want to consider that the child's respiratory and cardiovascular systems may be compromised and unstable. The child may have decreased vital capacity, restricted lung disease, an impaired cough, and the potential for developing pneumonia (Schwartz, 2008). Referrals to a pulmonologist, respiratory therapist, and pediatric cardiologist are in order if the respiratory muscles are weak, ventilation becomes necessary, cardiomyopathy develops, or there are cardiac arrhythmias.

Nutrition that enhances health and prevents obesity is important. Nurses should monitor growth, health, weight profile, and development carefully. Referral to nutrition services is recommended.

There are safety concerns for the child with progressive MD. Home and school environmental safety precautions are important to prevent falls and injury. Wheelchair accessibility may be necessary. Car seats offer needed neck support, and wheelchair-accessible vans augment travel and independence (Battista, 2010). A special parking permit and home adaptations for wheelchairs can be handled by a social worker or nurse case manager.

Immunizations are vital, and there are no restrictions. Precautions should be taken in children receiving high doses of corticosteroids. As is true of other neuromuscular disorders, dental care may require adaptive equipment.

Corrective orthopedic surgery may be needed to improve quality of life in some cases. Tendon contracture releases and corrective joint surgery may improve function. Sometimes a child may have painful muscle and tendon contractures. Percutaneous muscle release surgery may be indicated just for pain relief. Surgery for scoliosis may help correct progressive curvature of the spine. Assistive devices such as braces to offer support for weak muscles and therapy for the lower extremities may provide stretching of muscles and tendons and slow the progression of contractures. Canes, walkers, and wheelchairs can maintain mobility and independence.

Occupational and physical therapy

The goal of therapy is to maintain independence as long as possible. Physical therapy, occupational therapy, orthotic intervention, speech therapy, and orthopedic instruments such as wheelchairs and standing frames may be helpful. There is no specific treatment for any of the forms of MD. Physical therapy is helpful to prevent contractures and maintain muscle tone. Orthoses and orthopedic appliances can be used for support. Night splints and passive or active stretching exercises should be performed routinely. Aqua therapy may relieve joint pressure and encourage easier extremity movement.

Occupational therapy assists children with MD to engage in activities of daily living such as self-feeding and self-care. Leisure activities can be pursued at the most independent level possible. This may be achieved with use of adaptive equipment or the utilization of energy conservation techniques. Occupational therapy may implement changes to a person's environment, both at home or work, to increase the individual's function and accessibility. Occupational therapists also address the psychosocial changes and cognitive decline that may accompany MD; they also provide support and education about the disease to the family and individual.

Speech and language therapy

Children with Duchene's MD have high rates of speech and language delays. Therefore, speech therapy should be started early to help improve communication skills (Battista, 2010). Teachers should be aware of potential or actual problems with writing, typing, and talking. Adaptations may be necessary. Children with cognitive deficits may need special education classes.

Social work and psychology

Children with MD and their families will need psychological support. Support groups for families coping with MD can provide a forum to share common problems and help locate sources of social and medical support in the area where the families live. Adaptation at home, at school, and in the workplace will enhance the likelihood that individuals with MD will lead fulfilling lives. The Muscular Dystrophy Association is an excellent resource for families, friends, and teachers.

TRAUMATIC BRAIN INJURY

Traumatic brain injury (TBI) results from a severe insult to the brain caused by a traumatic force such as a direct blow to the head during a motor vehicle accident. The injury can be inflicted by a penetrating object or forces of deceleration, acceleration, a coup-contrecoup injury, or rotational trauma. Deceleration occurs when the head hits an immovable object. Acceleration occurs when a moving object strikes the head. A coup injury happens when the brain strikes the cranium on the side of impact, and a contrecoup injury happens when the brain rebounds and strikes the cranium on the contralateral side. Rotational trauma occurs when the brain is twisted during deceleration or acceleration.

Etiologies

The most common causes of brain injury in children result from traumatic falls, motor vehicle accidents, bicycle accidents, and child abuse. Head injuries are classified by severity (mild, moderate, and severe), as open or closed injuries, and as focal or diffuse. Penetrating wounds to the head often cause open injuries, whereas non-penetrating wounds such as contusions and hematomas are more likely to cause closed head injuries. Focal brain trauma is localized to one area of the brain and diffuse injuries happen when there is widespread brain damage.

Presenting signs and symptoms

Presenting signs and symptoms vary depending on the severity and type of head injury. Sometimes in a mild injury with concussion, such as from a minor sports injury, the trauma may not be recognized immediately. Therefore, obtaining a thorough history of the incident is crucial.

Prognosis

The length of time the child experiences coma is often associated with the severity of neurologic impairment. A coma lasting longer than seven days is more likely to result in some degree of cognitive dysfunction.

In addition to cognitive dysfunction, other neurologic dysfunction may include posttraumatic seizures, hydrocephalus, abnormal motor and sensory abilities, impaired respiratory function, speech and language deficits, endocrine dysfunction, and psychological or social problems.

Common pharmacologic and non-pharmacologic therapies

Therapies will be dictated by the extent of trauma and the subsequent associated problems. As mentioned earlier in this chapter, primary healthcare should address the needs of each individual child. Appropriate referrals to specialized care and rehabilitation are of utmost importance for recovery and long-term outcomes.

Posttraumatic seizures, which may require care by a pediatric neurologist, may respond to anticonvulsant medication. Anticonvulsants may be prescribed prophylactically for a period of time and then may be discontinued if chronic seizures do not develop. Cognitive dysfunction may require special education; school-based support; and referrals to physical, occupation, and speech therapy.

Some children with TBI experience endocrine dysfunction such as hypothyroidism or precocious puberty, which may be secondary to trauma to the hypothalamus or pituitary gland. These children need to be followed by pediatric endocrinology. Motor disabilities resulting from severe trauma may include spasticity, or other types of movement disorders such as those outlined in the discussion of CP, muscle and tendon contractures, paralysis and speech disorders. Impaired respiratory function may necessitate ventilation and respiratory support initially, or even chronically in some cases.

Roles of nursing

Nurses play a key role in monitoring and addressing the affects of traumatic brain injury. A child's growth and development should be monitored closely. Developmental progress and milestone attainment can be indicative of the long-term outcomes of brain trauma. Attention deficits, memory problems, and loss of verbal skills are not uncommon. Emotional assessment tools such as the revised Minnesota Multiphasic Personality Inventory (Tellegen et al., 2003) can be used to assess potential changes in mood or personality. Emotional disturbances such as depression and anxiety are common. Children with brain trauma may suffer from persistent irritability and undergo personality changes. Older children may exhibit cognitive deficits and poor social behavior judgment, and impaired self-restraint. Traditional approaches to problem behavior may be unsuccessful with these children if cognitive and social perceptual deficits exist.

Occupational and physical therapy

Rehabilitation focuses on avoiding secondary complications, teaching children to manage their disabilities, and enhancing their psychological adjustment. Children often recover normal function of motor skills after a head injury, but in some children motor dysfunction such as ataxia, tremor, hemiparesis, or spasticity may persist. Severe motor impairments may require adaptive equipment such as walkers, wheelchairs, or other technological devices such as specialized computers and electronic switches.

Speech and language therapy

Because of oral and motor problems, some children will exhibit signs of speech and/or language difficulties that persist over time after a head injury. Dysnomia may occur, making it difficult to retrieve a specific name of an object or person, particularly during a demanding situation. Dysarthria, which is slow, poorly articulated speech, is also common. Written language skills may be impaired because of underlying language deficits or motor dysfunction. Speech therapy may improve communication skills and provide some positive adaptations to these changes.

SPINAL CORD INJURY

Spinal cord injuries (SCI) affect between four and five million Americans per year. Most spinal cord injuries occur between the ages of 16 and 30, and about 79% of those who experience spinal cord injuries are male (Brain and Spinal Cord Organization, 2011).

Etiologies

National data indicate that about 20% (2,200) of all new traumatic SCI cases per year (about 11,000) occur in people under age 20, with about 2%–5% (250–500) of cases occurring in children from birth to 15 years, and

14%–18% (1500–2000) found in the 16–20 age group (Jackson, Dijkers, DeVivo, & Poczatek, 2004). These statistics do not include children with non-traumatic injuries from medical conditions such as transverse myelitis, spinal cord infarct and spinal tumors.

According to the NINDS (2011), spinal cord injury usually begins with a sudden, traumatic blow to the spine that fractures or dislocates vertebrae. The damage begins at the moment of injury when displaced bone fragments, disc material, or ligaments bruise or tear into spinal cord tissue. Most injuries to the spinal cord do not completely sever the cord. An injury is more likely to cause fractures and compression of the vertebrae, which then crush and destroy the axons, extensions of nerve cells that carry signals up and down the spinal cord between the brain and the rest of the body. An injury to the spinal cord can damage a few, many, or almost all of these axons. Some injuries will allow almost complete recovery. Other injuries will result in complete paralysis.

Prognosis

SCIs are classified as either complete or incomplete. In an incomplete injury, the ability of the spinal cord to convey messages to and from the brain is not completely lost. Children with an incomplete injury retain some motor or sensory function below the injury. A complete injury is indicated by a total lack of sensory and motor function below the level of injury. Children who survive an SCI will most likely have medical complications such as chronic pain and bladder and bowel dysfunction, along with an increased susceptibility to respiratory and heart problems. Successful recovery depends upon how well these chronic conditions are treated over the long term (NINDS, 2011).

Presenting signs and symptoms

After an injury, the degree of SCI is usually diagnosed with an MRI. MRI uses a powerful magnetic field, radio frequency pulses, and a computer to produce detailed pictures of organs, soft tissues, bone, and virtually all other internal body structures. The images can then be examined on a computer monitor. An MRI of the spine shows the anatomy of the vertebrae that make up the spine, the discs, spinal cord, and spaces between the vertebrae through which nerves pass. Currently, MRI is the most sensitive imaging test of the spine.

Common pharmacologic and non-pharmacologic therapies

NINDS conducts spinal cord research in its laboratories at the National Institutes of Health (NIH) and also supports additional research through grants to major medical institutions across the country. Advances in research are giving medical professionals and patients hope that repairing an injured spinal cord is a reachable goal. Advances in basic research are also being matched by progress in clinical research, especially in understanding the kinds of physical rehabilitation that work best to restore function. Some of the more promising rehabilitation techniques are helping SCI patients become more mobile (NINDS, 2011).

Roles of healthcare providers

After a child's medical status stabilizes, a continued focus on physical needs is the priority. There are many considerations for professionals and families caring for children with SCIs. The most important and troublesome problems are discussed in this section. Autonomic dysreflexia can occur with a distended or irritated urinary bladder. Autonomic dysreflexia is an acute elevation of blood pressure associated with a pounding headache, diaphoresis, facial flushing, nasal congestion, piloerection, and sometimes bradycardia. Treatment involves slowly emptying the distended bladder.

Urologic complications are common. SCI that affects the peripheral nerves will cause a flaccid urinary bladder, often called a neurogenic bladder. Intermittent urinary catheterization may be necessary. Urinary tract infections can result from poor perineal hygiene, contaminated equipment, and poor catheterization technique. Another complication of SCI is formation of renal stones. Stones form because of bone demineralization due to non-weight bearing and to calcium excretion through the urinary tract.

Autonomic dysreflexia can occur with fecal impaction. Other complications are paralytic ileus and bowel problems due to a state of atrophy of the small bowel with an absence of normal peristaltic movement. Defection reflexes will return if the SCI is above the sacral segments. Gastrointestinal bleeding may occur because of an increased release of steroids (from prolonged steroid therapy) or from increased hydrochloric acid production in the stomach. A bowel management program to prevent constipation is essential. Sufficient dietary fiber and fluids are needed to produce well-formed stools. Some children will require medications such as the bowel cleanser and laxative polyethylene glycol (MiraLAX®) to achieve smooth, regular bowel evacuation.

Drugs that can interfere with defecation are the anticholinergic medication oxybutynin chloride (Ditropan®), often used for urinary incontinence; ferrous sulfate (elemental iron) for anemia; narcotic analgesics such as hydrocodone; and mood elevators such as selective serotonin reuptake inhibitors. Some antibiotics such as cephalosporins and antacids such as milk of magnesium may contribute to diarrhea.

Ongoing skin care and monitoring are of the utmost importance because children with SCI are at high risk for skin breakdown. Individuals with SCI do not perspire below the level of the spinal injury in response to high environmental temperature. They do sweat profusely due to medical complications, however. The skin must stay clean and dry to prevent maceration and the risk of developing skin breakdown and decubitus ulcers. The loss or lack of sensation presents many hazards. The areas of the body that are especially vulnerable are the ischial tuberosities, sacrum, coccyx, greater trochanters, ankles, heels, and elbows. An infected decubitus can also trigger autonomic dysreflexia. Meticulous skin care using cleansing agents, antibacterial agents, topical anti-inflammatory drugs, chemical debriding agents, and occlusive dressings to wounds is imperative. Protective gel pads; cushions; bed coverings; and elbow, heel, and ankle pads may all work to promote healthy skin integrity. If serious skin breakdown does occur, referral to a wound expert is recommended. Potential environmental hazards include hot water, heaters, water pipes, cigarettes, and the rays of the sun. Lack of proprioception, loss of mobility, and impaired circulation all continue to be risk factors for problems. A routine turning schedule, muscle and tendon stretching, and active or passive range of motion exercises are crucial.

Some children will experience SCI-related pain that results from spinal deformities, postural instability, long bone fractures, hip dislocation, pressure sores, urinary tract infections, and spasticity (Massagli & Engel, 2006). Nurses should be familiar with pain behaviors and various pain assessment tools for younger children such as the Wong-Baker Faces Scale (Wong et al., 2001) (Figure 2.1) or the Visual Analogue Scale (Huskisson, 1974) for older children.

Medications for spasticity include Baclofen, a GABA Beta receptor agonist; Tizanidine, an alpha adrenergic receptor agonist; Dantrolenesodium, which blocks calcium release from the sacroplasmic reticulum; and diazepam, which facilitates GABA alpha mediated inhibition in the central nervous system. Diazepam has rapid onset and relief of spasticity, but should not be used as a first-line therapy because of addiction potential.

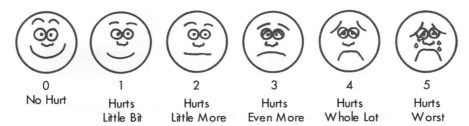

| 0 | 1 | 2 | 3 | 4 | 5 |
| No Hurt | Hurts Little Bit | Hurts Little More | Hurts Even More | Hurts Whole Lot | Hurts Worst |

Figure 2.1 The FACES Pain Rating Scale is a pain assessment tool that is appropriate for younger or cognitively impaired children. Wong, D.L, et al: Wong's Essentials of Pediatric Nursing, ed. 6, St. Louis, 2001, p. 1301. Copyrighted by Mosby, Inc. Reprinted with permission.

Occupational, physical, and speech therapies

Children with non-traumatic SCIs need similar rehabilitation to those with traumatic SCI (National Spinal Cord Injury Association, 2011). For specifics, refer to earlier sections of this chapter.

Social work and psychology

Reactions to now being disabled are often consistent with the stages of grieving over loss. Initially the child and family experience shock and denial, anger and depression. Hopefully, acceptance and adaptation begin to occur as the child remolds his or her self-concept to include the disability. Developmental stages of childhood may be affected. A sense of trust, autonomy, motivation, and self-identity may be compromised. Family members may experience hopelessness, powerlessness, frustration, guilt, depression, and anxiety. Role changes, economic stress, and physical exhaustion may all lead to overwhelming family turmoil.

According to Massagli (2005), positive outcomes and life satisfaction are strongly related to functional independence and involvement in community. Rehabilitation prepares families for the future by maximizing education, participation, and independence. Massagli reported that a parent once told her that "the most valuable thing she learned when her son was in rehabilitation was that once the physical barriers were removed, there was so much he was still able to do." This mother made their home and transportation accessible to her son and advocated for him in school and sports. Her son has become a successful college student and competitive wheelchair athlete.

Job and vocational planning within the child's capacity to perform and the necessary educational requirements for success are important. The child also needs a sense of safety, love and belonging, self-respect and acceptance, socialization, and achievement and recognition. Enhancing the child's self-esteem is important. Some children may have a sleep pattern disturbance and ineffective coping skills and impulsivity. They will need ongoing therapy for issues such as these.

In the older child, sexual function will become a major issue. Sexual health should be integral to rehabilitation. Body image and self-esteem are often affected by a SCI, and sexual relationships and developing intimate partner relationships may be difficult (Cardenas, Hoffman, & Stockman, 2006). Sexually active males with an SCI can impregnate a female, and females of childbearing age with SCI run the risk of pregnancy because SCI does not affect fertility. Need for birth control, prevention of sexually transmitted infections, and concerns for contracting and transmitting human papilloma virus and subsequent cervical dysplasia are no different than for people without a SCI. Birth control pills may increase the risk of thrombophlebitis in women with an SCI (Hickey, 2006). Information on sexuality is important. Females may be concerned that they cannot bear children. Boys may fear they may not be able to sustain an erection or have an ejaculation. Education about these and other aspects of sexual education should be central to any comprehensive program for children with SCI.

CHILDREN WITH DEAFNESS AND HEARING IMPAIRMENT

Each year 24,000 children are born with a hearing loss in the United States (US Department of Education, 2006). The majority of these children are born to parents who have normal hearing. Congenital deafness occurs 2 to 3 times per 1000 births (Vohr, 2003). At least 50% of early-onset deafness is genetic and not associated with syndromes (Palmer, Lueddeke, & Zhou, 2009). Universal newborn hearing screening programs and advances in hearing technology have enhanced early treatment options for families (Yoshinaga-Itano, 2003). Many states now require that hospitals screen newborns at birth for possible hearing loss.

Etiology of deafness

Causes of hearing loss later in childhood include genetic factors, illness, and trauma (Korver et al., 2011). The degree of hearing loss can vary from mild to profound, including deafness. There are four different kinds of hearing loss. A conductive hearing loss is caused by diseases or obstructions in the outer or middle ear. A sensorineural loss is a condition where the delicate sensory hair cells of the inner ear are damaged. A mixed hearing loss is a combination of the two. A central loss results from damage to the nerves of the central nervous system.

Conductive hearing loss results from a problem in the outer or middle ear, such as wax buildup, rupture of the eardrum, or repeated infections. It is usually possible to treat conductive hearing loss with medication or surgery (Kliegman, Behrman, Jenson, & Stanton, 2007). Causes of conductive hearing loss in infants include abnormalities in the structure of the ear canal or middle ear or from ear wax impaction. Ear infections, especially recurring infections, foreign objects in the ear, injury, eardrum perforation, or tumors can also cause this type of hearing loss.

Sensorineural hearing loss results from a problem with the inner ear. The inner ear is responsible for sending signals to the auditory nerve. Causes of sensorineural hearing loss include exposure to certain intrauterine toxic

COMMON PHYSICAL OR SENSORY DISABILITIES

chemicals or medications, genetic disorders such as Down syndrome, and prenatal infection such as cytomegalovirus or rubella in the first trimester of pregnancy. Postnatal infections such as bacterial meningitis and congenital structural deformities of the inner ear can be causes. Noise-induced hearing loss is a major cause of deafness and hearing impairment in the United States, one becoming more common among children with the increase in exposure to portable music players (Daniel, 2007).

Hearing-impaired children lag behind children of normal hearing in receptive vocabulary and the ability to learn new words (Pittman, Lewis, Hoover, & Stelmachowicz, 2005). Impairment in language and communication development may play an important role in the emergence of behavioral problems in young children, and there are strong links between language delays and behavior problems. Studies show that children diagnosed with language disorders demonstrate a higher incidence of behavior problems than their nondisabled peers, and children diagnosed with behavior problems demonstrate a higher incidence of language disorders (Barker et al., 2009).

Presenting signs and symptoms

Signs of hearing loss in infants vary by age. A neonate with a hearing loss may not be startled by a loud noise. Older infants, who should normally be responding to familiar voices, may show no reaction when spoken to. Children should be using single words by age 15 months and simple two-word sentences by age 2. If they do not reach these milestones, hearing loss may be the cause.

Some children may not be diagnosed until they are in school, even if they were born with a hearing loss. Inattention and falling behind in class work may be the result of an undiagnosed hearing impairment. A physical exam with detailed otoscopy may reveal problems such as bone deformation, perforated eardrum, or signs of genetic changes that may cause hearing loss.

Hearing loss results in a child's inability to hear sounds in ranges that children with normal hearing can readily hear. Subjective and objective audiological tests exist; the tests used depend upon the child's age and development. Two common tests are used to screen newborn infants for hearing loss. The auditory brain stem response test uses electrodes to determine how the auditory nerve reacts to sound. The otoacoustic emissions test involves microphones placed into the infant's ears to detect nearby sounds. The sounds echo in the ear canal. If there is no echo, it is a sign of hearing loss.

Older infants and young children can be taught to respond to sounds through play. These tests, known as visual response audiometry and play audiometry, can better determine the child's range of hearing. Diagnostic tests that may be performed include audiometry (an electronic hearing test) and an auditory response test. The caloric test measures the degree to which the vestibular system is responsive and how symmetric the responses are between the left and right ears. A computerized tomography scan of the head is done if an underlying tumor or fracture is suspected. An MRI of the ear or head may be performed if a tumor or stroke is suspected. Tympanometry tests the condition of the middle ear and mobility of the eardrum. An X-ray of the head may be done if cranial structural problems may be a cause for hearing loss.

Prognosis

If a hearing deficit is not diagnosed early in childhood, the child's development may be halted (Hempel, 2006). Effects of deafness on language and learning can be devastating (Watkin et al., 2007). Sensorineural deafness may be inherited or acquired. If inherited, deafness may be a part of a number of congenital syndromes. Acquired deafness may occur in the prenatal, perinatal, or postnatal stages of development (Hempel). Sound conduction deafness can be temporary or permanent. The prognosis for the child with hearing loss depends on the cause and severity of the hearing loss. There is no cure for sensorineural hearing loss. Children with this type of hearing loss may benefit from hearing aids or a cochlear implant. Advances in hearing aid technology and speech therapy allow many children to develop normal language skills at the same age as their peers with normal hearing. Infants with profound hearing loss can still fare well with the proper support. Complications such as delayed speech and problems with receptive language (understanding words) and the ability to make friends can hamper the child's development. Emotional problems due to feelings of isolation and falling behind in school can occur. If hearing loss is the result of a disease or syndrome that affects other parts of the body, other medical problems can appear.

Over 30 states in the United States have mandatory hearing screenings of newborns (Kaneshiro, 2010). Early treatment of hearing loss can allow many infants to develop normal language skills without delay. In infants born with hearing loss, treatments should start as early as possible, preferably by 6 months of age. Treatment depends on the child's overall health and cause of hearing loss. Treatment may involve surgery, medications, speech therapy, learning sign language, or receiving a cochlear implant.

Common pharmacologic and non-pharmacologic therapies

Many services are now available to help children with a hearing impairment. Children with hearing loss in the past struggled for years with challenges of acquiring spoken language. Now children have more options for achieving speech and language.

Cochlear implants especially have become widely embraced as an aid to exposing the deaf child's auditory system to a quality of sound experience not available with hearing aids alone (Nicholas & Geers, 2007). Improvements in speech-enhancing strategies include cochlear implants, which are particularly helpful in understanding speech. Children with cochlear implants represent a unique population of individuals who have undergone variable amounts of auditory deprivation before being able to hear (Litovsky, Johnstone, & Godar, 2006a). In most cochlear implant users, speech reception in a noisy or complex environment is not optimal. Children can benefit from wearing two hearing devices (one in both ears) compared with a single device in one ear (Litovsky, Johnstone, & Godar, 2006b).

Hearing aids make sounds louder in the ranges needed, which are dictated by the child's hearing loss. Hearing aids operate on very small batteries; they collect sounds, make them louder, and then transfer the sounds to the ear canal. When a child has a hearing loss, it is important to fit the child with hearing aids as early as possible because children begin identifying sounds and learning language in the first months of life. Hearing aids can give children the opportunity to hear and learn language in much the same way as children with normal hearing. Even infants can wear hearing aids. Each hearing aid is selected for, and fitted to, a child's individual needs. An audiologist will determine what type of hearing aid is best for a child.

If a child has not benefited from hearing aids after wearing them for several months, the child may be a candidate for a cochlear implant, a device surgically implanted in the ear. Unlike hearing aids, a cochlear implant does not make sound louder but bypasses the damaged parts of the ear and sends an electronic signal directly along the auditory nerve to the brain. Cochlear implants are approved by the Food and Drug Administration for children 12 months of age or older. Good candidates for a cochlear implant are those children who have a severe hearing loss and have received little or no benefit from wearing hearing aids.

Role of nursing

Nurses are in a position to assure that infants are screened for hearing loss even before leaving the hospital or in early infancy. Once a hearing loss has been suspected or detected, families will need community resources to assist them in securing proper care for their children. Depending on the cause of the hearing loss, some children with global health problems such as congenital syndromes will need additional healthcare by specialists. Hearing loss may be only one of many problems for these children.

Children with sensory disabilities such as blindness and deafness are at an increased risk of injuries as a result of difficulties identifying and responding to hazards in the environment. One study (Mann, Zhou, McKee, & McDermott, 2007) found that children with hearing loss were twice as likely to be treated for emergent injuries as their nondisabled peers.

Modifiable health behaviors that increase the risk of hearing loss in children should begin early in childhood to prevent or delay the onset of hearing impairment (Daniel, 2007). Wearing hearing protection when operating machinery and avoiding loud music are behaviors that nurses can promote in their communities and in clinical practices. Chung, Des Roches, Meunier, & Eavey (2005) found that most teenagers responding to Internet-based survey questions about general health did not consider hearing loss to be a major health concern.

Vaccinations such as the meningococcal vaccine that protect against bacteria that cause meningitis can help prevent hearing loss and reduce the risk of disease in a child with a cochlear implant. Children with cochlear implants may be at a higher risk for bacterial meningitis (O'Handley, Tobin, & Tagge, 2007).

Occupational and physical therapy

The role of occupational therapists may be crucial in children with hearing impairment because schooling and eventually vocational pursuits will require accommodations for most children. Therapists may be involved in early intervention, community-based programs, preschool and school programs for hearing-impaired children, outpatient clinics, rehabilitation settings, or community mental health programs.

Speech and language therapy

Speech therapy has a primary role in children with deafness and hearing loss. The auditory-verbal approach teaches children to make effective use of their residual hearing either via hearing aids or a cochlear implant. Therapists work one-on-one with the child to teach him or her to rely only on listening skills. Because parent involvement is an important part of the auditory-verbal approach, therapists also partner with parents and caregivers to provide them with the skills they need to help the child become an auditory communicator. In this approach, neither speech reading nor the use of sign language is taught.

In cued speech, children learn to see movements that the mouth makes when talking. This is combined with eight hand shapes, called *cues*, indicating groups of consonants, and four positions around the face, indicating vowel sounds. The hand cues help children determine what sounds are being voiced.

There are two basic types of sign language. Signed Exact English (SEE) is an artificial language that follows the grammatical structure of English. American Sign Language (ASL) is a language that follows its own grammatical rules. It is often taught as the child's first language. English may then be taught as a second language.

In total communication the above-mentioned methods are combined. Children learn a form of sign communication and also incorporate finger spelling, speech reading, speaking, and either hearing aids or cochlear implants.

Social work and psychology

Families of children with special needs such as visual and hearing impairment often have responsibilities and face challenges over and above those of children without special needs. These responsibilities may include advocating for their children, making decisions about the healthcare of their children, and participating in their children's education. Parents may try to compensate for their children when they are not able to achieve typical developmental achievements (Anderson, 2009). Families will generate opportunities for their children to socialize, steer them through a maze of healthcare encounters, plot out a way for them to get an appropriate education, and investigate services that are available to them. Coordination of supportive health care, school, and community partnerships is often inadequate (Anderson). Almost 30% of mothers of children with special needs report having to reduce or stop employment to care for their children (US Department of Health and Human Services, 2011).

Services available to help children who have hearing loss, including deafness, are numerous in some areas of the United States and other developed countries. Infants and toddlers may be eligible for state Early Intervention programs. Children from ages 3 to 18 may benefit from special education and related services at school (US Department of Education, 2006). However, many hearing-impaired children live in areas without specialized services, and these services do not even exist in many countries.

CHILDREN WITH BLINDNESS AND VISUAL IMPAIRMENT

The World Health Organization (2011) defines blindness as the best corrected vision in the better eye of less than 3/60 or a visual field ≤10°, whereas severe visual impairment is defined as the best corrected visual acuity in the better eye of 3/60 or more, but less than 6/60 or a visual field ≤20°. Legal blindness can be defined as the level of blindness that makes a child eligible for social support and financial benefits. Blindness occurs in about 3% of the world's population. In many cases it can be prevented with adequate nutrition and good healthcare.

Etiology

Vitamin A deficiency, neonatal eye infections, congenital cataracts and congenital glaucoma account for most cases of childhood blindness worldwide (World Health Organization, 2011). Poor hygiene, overcrowding, ultraviolet radiation, diabetes mellitus, drugs, nutritional deficiency, heredity, ethnic background, and consanguinity are other risk factors for vision loss. Children born with albinism may be legally blind but have some vision. Eye injuries, most often occurring in people under age 30, are the leading cause of monocular blindness (vision loss in one eye) in the United States.

Other causes of blindness are eye malformations, retinopathy of prematurity, trauma, and tumors such as a retinal blastoma. Retinopathy of prematurity occurs almost exclusively in premature infants who received oxygen therapy to treat respiratory distress syndrome.

Less severe and more common visual impairments include strabismus, nystagmus, and amblyopia. Strabismus is a condition in which the eyes are not properly aligned with each other. Nystagmus is involuntary eye movement. Amblyopia is a condition in which visual stimulation either fails to transmit or is poorly transmitted through the optic nerve and brain. Children will have poor or dim vision. Amblyopia normally affects only one eye, but it is possible to have the condition in both eyes, resulting in a lack of clear vision. Detection of the condition in early childhood increases the chance of successful treatment (American Optometrist Association, 2011).

Presenting signs and symptoms

Elicitation of a gray or white reflex on retinoscopy of the infant or young child requires immediate referral to an opthamologist. In addition, a visually impaired infant may not respond to patterns and bright colors in the way that non–visually impaired infants do. The young infant with visual impairment may be delayed in milestones such as demonstration of social smiling and may not engage in reciprocal attachment behaviors that require reading of body language.

COMMON PHYSICAL OR SENSORY DISABILITIES

Prognosis

The prognosis for the child with visual impairment depends on a number of factors already mentioned, including type and severity of insult and available services.

Common pharmacologic and non-pharmacologic therapies

Treatment of visual impairment should try to address all the disabling conditions; therefore a multidisciplinary team approach is essential. The primary ways for the blind child to explore the world are through touch and sound. Parents should be encouraged to give their child toys that enhance tactile awareness. Standing and walking may be difficult initially because the child lacks visual perception. Gross motor development may be slower, but will improve over time. Touching and physical affection are important. Parents should talk to their children, explaining and visually describing their surroundings.

Role of nursing

The needs of children with visual impairment vary depending on the health of the individual child and the cause of blindness. If visual acuity is less than 20/200 with corrective lenses, the child is legally blind. With 20/2000 vision the child can read large-print books, but totally blind children must rely on Braille or other aids. Nurses can discuss with parents the special needs their child may have.

If the child is admitted to the hospital for care, it is helpful if parents can stay with their child while the environment is still unfamiliar. Nurses should introduce themselves and address the child by name, so the child knows he or she is being spoken to, and should introduce the child to his or her roommates. The assessment should always include asking the parent or caregiver what the child is able to see because few children are totally blind. Being blind or vision-impaired does not mean the child cannot hear or understand what is being said. A good-bye when finished indicates when the nurse is leaving the room.

Leaving infants who are blind lying on their back for long periods, even though they may seem content, puts them at risk for sensory deprivation. Their lack of responsiveness must not be mistaken for deafness or intellectual handicap. Appropriate, consistent stimulation, such as soft talking and gentle touching, is imperative (Vision Australia, 2011). A blind infant learns about surroundings through mouthing, and later through tactile exploration. Ensuring that the infant has familiar and enjoyable toys within easy reach will help with stimulation. Toys should have varied textures, make interesting noises, and be safe and pleasant for the mouth.

A toddler should be able to explore the environment freely and as independently as possible. It is important that caregivers explain what is being done and describe new surroundings and situations. A hands-on approach is important in the introduction of new objects. For example, the caregiver should show children where their food or drink is on the tray and how to open containers.

As children get older it is important that they wear protective eyewear while engaging in activities and wear light reflective sunglasses outdoors so that existing vision is preserved. Avoiding unnecessary furniture moving and being aware of any possible obstacles or hazards such as sharp corners and extension cords will promote safety in the home, hospital, and school. Encouraging children to practice their abilities and engage in age-appropriate individual and group play is recommended (Vision Australia, 2011). Color contrast can be important for children who are vision-impaired. Other recommendations made by Vision Australia are the following:

- Read aloud menu items and let the patient choose his or her meal.

- Tell children when their meal has arrived and where their food tray is placed.

- Assist younger children with removing packaging from items.

- Ask older children if they need assistance with their meal, rather than just offering to cut their food.

- Provide any hot drinks in non-spill containers and tell the patient where they are placed.

Occupational and physical therapy

Assistive technology for visually impaired children is continually improving. Voice recognition computer applications permit children to input instructions verbally. Computers convert printing into Braille. They produce voice messages, vocalize results of mathematical calculations, and interface to produce tactile digital information.

Communities are becoming more aware and accessible to visually impaired people. Children with severe visual impairment normally learn to type on a computer keyboard by the fourth grade. Books on tape can be found in bookstores and public libraries. It is important that families have the equipment necessary for the child's learning benefits and independence.

Safety issues in cooking and meal preparation can be addressed by occupational therapy. Information about activities such as grocery shopping; kitchen accommodations; selection of appliances; and techniques for measuring, pouring, and cooking can be promoted in older children to prepare them for adulthood.

Orientation and mobility services and instructions are a part of rehabilitation and education that children, parents, and teachers can benefit from in order for the blind child to travel safely and be more independent. Components of orientation and mobility instruction are engaging in sensory training, developing good spatial and environmental concepts, building confidence, training in functional travel, learning self-protection techniques, discovering sight-guided techniques, becoming skilled in independent travel, and gaining knowledge in safely and efficiently using available public transportation (Board of Education & Services for the Blind, 2011).

Speech and language therapy

Children learn to speak by imitating mouth movements in addition to listening to sounds. Therefore, language development may be delayed in blind children. The blind child learns to speak using auditory means only. Speech may be accomplished but there may be less body and facial expressions. A speech therapy assessment and therapy are prudent.

REFERENCES

American Academy of Pediatrics. (2011). http://www.aap.org

American Optometrist Association. (2011). http://www.aoa.org

American Academy for Cerebral Palsy and Developmental Medicine. (2011). www.aacpdm.org

Anderson, L.S. (2009). Mothers of children with special health care needs: Documenting the experience of their children's care in the school setting. *Journal of School Nursing*, *25*(5), 342–351.

Barker, D.H., Quittner, A.L., Fink, N.E., et al. (2009). Predicting behavior problems in deaf and hearing children: The influences of language, attention, and parent–child communication. *Developmental Psychopathology*, *21*(2), 373–392.

Battista, V. (2010). Muscular dystrophy. Duchenne. In P.J. Allen, J.A. Vessey, & N.A. Schapiro (Eds.), *Primary care of the child with a chronic condition* (5th ed.) (pp. 654–670). St. Louis, MO: Mosby.

Bell, K.R., Pepping, M., & Dikmen, S. (2006). Rehabilitation after traumatic brain injury. In L.R. Robinson (Ed.), *Traumatic rehabilitation* (pp. 91–114) Philadelphia:, PA: Lippincott, Williams, & Wilkins.

Blosser, C.G. (2009). Eye disorders. In C.E. Burns, A.M. Dunn, M.A. Brady, N.B. Starr, & C.G. Blosser (Eds.), *Pediatric primary care* (4th ed.) (pp. 673–704). St. Louis, MO: Saunders.

Board of Education and Services for the Blind. (2011). *BESB: Orientation and Mobility Services*. http://www.ct.gov

Brain and Spinal Cord Organization. (2011). http://www.brainandspinalcord.org/

Broder, K.R., Cortese, M.M., Iskander, J., et al. (2006). Preventing tetanus, diphtheria, and pertussis among adolescents: Use of tetanus toxoid, reduced diphtheria toxoid, and acellular pertussis vaccines. Recommendations of the Advisory Committee on Immunization Practices. *MMWR Morbidity and Mortality Weekly Report, 55*(RR-3), 1–44.

Cameron, M., & Moran, P. (2009). Prenatal screening and diagnosis of neural tube defects. *Prenatal Diagnosis, 29*, 402.

Cardenas, D.D., Hoffman, J.M., & Stockman, P.L. (2006). *Spinal cord injury*. In L.R. Robinson, *Traumatic rehabilitation* (pp. 115–142). Philadelphia, PA: Lippincott, Williams, & Wilkins.

Casamassimo, P.S., Seale, N.S., & Ruehs, K. (2004). General dentists' perceptions of educational and treatment issues affecting access to care for children with special health care needs. *Journal of Dental Education, 68*(1), 23–28.

Centers for Disease Control and Prevention (CDC). (2008). Use of supplements containing folic acid among women of childbearing age – United States. *MMWR, 57*(01), 5–8.

Chung, J.H., Des Roches, C.M., Meunier, J., & Eavey, R.D. (2005). Evaluation of noise induced hearing loss in young people using a web-based survey technique. *Pediatrics, 115*(4), 861–867.

Daniel, E. (2007). Noise and hearing loss: A review. *Journal of School Health, 77*(5), 225–231.

Eyman, R.K., Grossman, H.J., Chaney, R.H., & Call, T.L. (1990). The life expectancy of profoundly handicapped people with mental retardation. *New England Journal of Medicine, 323*, 584–589.

Fiore, A.E., Wasley, A., & Bell, B.P. (2006). Prevention of hepatitis A through active or passive immunization. Recommendations of the Advisory Committee on Immunization Practices. *MMWR Morbidity and Mortality Weekly Report, 55*(RR-7), 1–23.

Frankenburg, W.K., & Dobbs, J.B. (1967). The Denver Developmental Screening Test. *Journal of Pediatrics, 71*(71): 181–191.

Harris, S.R. (2009). Listening to parents' concerns: Three case examples of infants with developmental motor delays. *Pediatric Physical Therapy, 21*, 269–274.

Hempel, J.M. (2006). Diagnosing hearing impairment in children. *MMW – Fortschritte der Medizin, 148*(19), 26–30.

Hickey, J.V. (2006). Vertebral and spinal cord injuries. In J.V. Hickey, *The clinical practice of neurological and neurosurgical nursing* (5th ed) (pp. 407–450) Philadelphia, PA: Lippincott, Williams, & Wilkins.

Hochberg, L. (2009). *Prenatal screening and diagnosis of neural tube defects*. Retrieved from http://www.uptodate.com/index/home.html.

Huskisson, E.C. (1974). Measurement of pain. *The Lancet, 9*(2): 1127–1131.

Jackson, A.B., Dijkers, M., DeVivo, M.J., & Poczatek, R.B. (2004). A demographic profile of new traumatic SCIs: Change and stability over 30 years. *Archives of Physical Medicine and Rehabilitation, 85*, 1740–1748.

COMMON PHYSICAL OR SENSORY DISABILITIES

COMMON PHYSICAL OR SENSORY DISABILITIES

Jones, M.W., Morgan, E., & Shelton, J.E. (2007). Primary care of the child with cerebral palsy: A review of systems. *Journal of Pediatric Health Care, 21*(4), 226–237.

Kaneshiro, N.K. (2010). Hearing loss infants. US National Library of Medicine, NIH National Institute of Health. Retrieved from http://www.nlm.nih.gov/medlineplus/ency/article/007322.htm

King, W.M., Ruttencutter, R., Kissel, J.T., et al. (2007). Orthopedic outcomes of long-term daily corticosteroid treatment in Duchenne muscular dystrophy. *Neurology 68*, 1607–1613.

Kliegman, R.M., Behrman, R.E., Jenson, H.B., & Stanton, B.F. (2007). *Nelson textbook of pediatrics* (18th ed). Philadelphia, PA: Elsevier.

Korver, A.M., Admiraal, R.J., Kant, S.G., et al. (2011). Causes of permanent childhood hearing impairment. *The Laryngoscope, 121*(2), 409–416.

Lazzaretti, C.C., & Pearson, C. (2010). *Myelodysplasia*. In P.J. Allen, J.A. Vessey, & N.A. Schapiro (Eds.), Primary care of the child with a chronic condition (5th ed.) (pp. 671–685). St. Louis, MO: Mosby.

Litovsky, R.Y., Johnstone, P.M., & Godar, S.P. (2006a). Benefits of bilateral cochlear implants and/or hearing aids in children. *International Journal of Audiology, 45*(Suppl 1), S78–S91.

Litovsky, R.Y., Johnstone, P.M., Godar, S., Agrawal, et al. (2006b). Bilateral cochlear implants in children: Localization acuity measured with minimum audible angle. *Ear and Hearing, 27*(1), 43–59.

Mann, J.R., Zhou, L., McKee, M., & McDermott, S. (2007). Children with hearing loss and increased risk of injury. *Annals of Family Medicine, 5*(6), 528–533.

Massagli, T. (2005). SCI in children and teens. *Spinal Cord Injury Update, 14*(1), 1.

Massagli, T. & Engel, J.M. (2006). *Special consideration for pediatric patients with disability due to trauma*. In L.R. Robinson, *Traumatic rehabilitation* (pp. 291–311). Philadelphia, PA: Lippincott, Williams, & Wilkins.

Mayo Clinic. (2011). Muscular dystrophy. Retrieved from http://mayoclinic.com/health/muscular-dystrophy/DS00200

McGrath, J.M., & Hardy, W. (2011). The infant at risk. In S. Mattson & J.E. Smith, *Core Curriculum for Maternal-Newborn Nursing, (4th ed)* pp. 362–414. St. Louis, MO: Saunders Elsevier.

Mello, R.R., Silva, K.S., Rodriques, M.C., et al. (2009). Predictive factors for neuro-motor abnormalities at the corrected age of 12 months in very low birth weight premature infants. *Arq Neuropsiquiatr, 67*(2A), 235–241.

National Institute of Neurological Disorders and Stroke. (2012). Spinal cord injuries. National Institutes of Health. Retrieved from http://www.ninds.nih.gov/disorders/sci/sci.htm

Nehring, W.M. (2010). Cerebral palsy. In P.J. Allen, J.A. Vessey, & N.A. Schapiro, *Primary Care of the Child with a Chronic Condition (5th ed.)* pp. 326–346. St. Louis, MO: Mosby.

Newborg, J. (2004). *Battelle developmental inventory* (2nd ed). Scarborough, Ontario: Nelson Education.

Newman, C.J., Holenweg-Gross, C., Vuillerot, C., et al. (2010). Recent skin injuries in children with motor disabilities. *Achives in Dis Child, 95*(5), 387–390.

New York State Department of Health. Latex Allergy Information for Health Professionals. May 2012. Retrieved from http://www.health.ny.gov/publications/1453/

Nicholas, J.G., & Geers, A.E. (2007). Will they catch up? The role of age at cochlear implantation in the spoken language development of children with severe-profound hearing loss. *Journal of Speech, Language, and Hearing Research, 50*(4), 1048–1062.

Odding, E., Roebroeck, M.E., & Stam, H.J. (2006). The epidemiology of cerebral palsy: Incidence, impairments, and risk factors. *Disability & Rehabilitation, 28,* 183–191.

O'Handley, J.G., Tobin, E., & Tagge, B. (2007). Otorhinolaryngology. In R.E. Rakel (Ed.), *Textbook of family medicine* (7th ed.) (pp. 413–462). Philadelphia, PA: Saunders Elsevier.

O'Shea, T.M. (2008). Diagnosis, treatment, and prevention of cerebral palsy in near-term/term infants. *Clinical Obstetrics and Gynecology, 51*(4), 816–828.

Padmanabhan, R. (2006). Etiology, pathogenesis, and prevention of neural tube defects. *Congenital Anomalies, 46,* 66–67.

Palmer, C.G.S., Lueddeke, J.T., & Zhou, J. (2009). Factors influencing parental decision about genetics evaluation for their deaf or hard-of-hearing child. *Genetics in Medicine, 11*(4), 248.

Paneth, N. (2008). Establishing the diagnosis of cerebral palsy. *Clinical Obstetrics and Gynecology, 51*(4), 742–748.

Petersen-Smith, A.M., & McKenzie, S.B. (2009). *Ear disorders.* In C.E. Burns, A.M. Dunn, M.A. Brady, N.B. Starr, & C.G. Blosser (Eds.), *Pediatric primary care* (4th ed) pp. 705–726. St. Louis, MO: Saunders.

Pittman, A.L., Lewis, D.E., Hoover, B.M., & Stelmachowicz, P.G. (2005). Rapid word-learning in normal-hearing and hearing-impaired children. Effects of age, receptive vocabulary, and high-frequency amplification. *Ear and Hearing, 26*(6), 619–629.

Russman, B.S. (2004). Evaluation of the child with cerebral palsy. *Seminars in Pediatric Neurology, 11*(1), 47–57.

Sawin, K.J., Cox, A.W., & Metzger, S.G. (2010). *Transition to adulthood.* In P.J. Allen, J.A. Vessey, & N.A. Schapiro (Eds.), *Primary care of the child with a chronic condition* (5th ed.) pp. 60–73. St. Louis, MO: Mosby.

Schwartz, M.W. (Ed.). (2008). *The 5 minute pediatric consult.* Philadelphia, PA: Wolters Kluwer.

Spina Bifida Association. (2012). Retrieved from http://www.spinabifidaassociation .org.

Tecklin, J.S. (2008). *Pediatric physical therapy* (4th ed). Philadelphia, PA: Lippincott, Williams, & Wilkins.

Tellegen, A., Ben-Porath, Y.S., McNulty, J.L., Arbisi, P.A., Graham, J.R., & Kaemmer, B. (2003). *The MMPI-2 Restructured Clinical Scales: Development, validation, and interpretation.* Minneapolis: University of Minnesota Press.

United States Department of Education. (2006). *Opening doors: Technology and communication options for children with hearing loss.* P.O. Box 1398, Jessup, MD 20794.

United States Department of Health and Human Services. (2011). *Title V.* Maternal and Child Health Bureau. Health Resources and Services Administration.

United States Preventive Services Task Force. (2009). *Folic acid for the prevention of neural tube defects.* United States Preventive Services Task Force recommendation statement. Rockville, MD, http://www.annals.org/cgi/reprint/150/9/626.pdf

Vision Australia. (March 22, 2011). *Blindness and low vision services.* http://www .visionaustralia.org

Vohr, B. (2003). Infants and children with hearing loss-Part 2: Overview. *Mental Retardation and Developmental Disabilities Research Reviews, 9,* 218–219.

COMMON PHYSICAL OR SENSORY DISABILITIES

Waldman, H.B., Perlman, S.P., & Rader, R. (2010). The transition of children with disabilities to adulthood: What about dental care? *Journal of the American Dental Association, 141*(8), 937–938.

Watkin, P., McCann, D., Law, C., et al. (2007). Language ability in children with permanent hearing impairment: The influence of early management and family participation. *Pediatrics, 120*(3): e694–701.

Wiegerink, D., Roebroeck, M.E., Donkervoort, M., et al. (2006). Social and sexual relationships of adolescents and young adults with cerebral palsy: A review. *Clinical Rehabilitation, 20*(12), 1023–1031.

Wong, D.L., Hockenberry-Eaton, M., Wilson, D., et al. (2001). *Wong's essentials of pediatric nursing* (6th ed.) St. Louis, MO: Mosby.

World Health Organization. (2011). *Prevention of Blindness and Visual Impairment.* http://www.who.int/blindness/en/

Yoshinaga-Itano, C. (2003). Early intervention after universal neonatal hearing screening: Impact on outcomes. *Mental Retardation and Developmental Disabilities Research Reviews, 9*, 252–266.

ONLINE RESOURCES

American Society for Deaf Children
1-866-895-4206
717-703-0073 (V/TTY)
www.deafchildren.org

Child Development and Rehabilitation Center
Oregon Health & Science University
Portland, OR
http://www.ohsu.edu/xd/health/child-development-and-rehabilitation-center/index.cfm

Hydrocephalus Association
870 Market Street Suite 705
San Francisco, CA 94102
www.hydroassco.org

March of Dimes
1275 Mamaroneck Avenue
White Plains, NY 10605
http://www.marchofdimes.com

Muscular Dystrophy Association, USA
National Headquarters
3300 E. Sunrise Drive

Tucson, AZ 85718
http://www.mdausa.org/

The National Dissemination Center for Children with Disabilities
NICHCY
P.O. Box 1492
Washington, DC 20013
1-800-695-0285 (V/TTY)
www.nichcy.org

National Institute on Deafness and Other Communication Disorders
1-800-241-1044
1-800-241-1055 (TTY)
www.nidcd.nih.gov

National Spinal Cord Injury Association (NSCIA)
6701 Democracy Blvd, Suite 300-9
Bethesda, MD 20817
(800) 962-9629
http://www.spinalcord.org/

Spina Bifida Association
4590 MacArthur Blvd. NW, Suite 250
Washington, DC   20007-4266
http://www.spinabifidaassociation.org

United Cerebral Palsy Association Inc. (UCP)
1660 L St. NW, Suite 700
Washington, DC 20036–5602
http://www.ucpa.org

CHAPTER 3
COMMON DEVELOPMENTAL/ LEARNING DISABILITIES

Linda L. Eddy

Caring for Children with Special Healthcare Needs and Their Families: A Handbook for Healthcare Professionals, First Edition. Edited by Linda L. Eddy.
© 2013 John Wiley & Sons, Inc. Published 2013 by John Wiley & Sons, Inc.

This chapter will examine common features of the following intellectual, developmental, and/or learning disabilities often encountered in children and adolescents: (a) attention-deficit/hyperactivity disorder, (b) intellectual disability with Down Syndrome as exemplar, and (c) pervasive developmental delay (autism and its variants). The focus will be on possible etiologies, presenting signs and symptoms, diagnostic tests, common therapies, and roles of nursing and other healthcare providers.

THE CHILD WITH ATTENTION DEFICIT/HYPERACTIVITY DISORDER

Definition and presenting signs and symptoms

Symptoms of attention deficit/hyperactivity disorder (ADHD) include difficulty staying focused and paying attention, difficulty controlling behavior, and hyperactivity. According to the *Diagnostic and Statistical Manual of Mental Disorders (2000) (DSM-IV-TR)*, ADHD has three subtypes: (a) Predominantly hyperactive-impulsive in which most symptoms are in the hyperactivity-impulsivity categories, and fewer than six symptoms of inattention are present; (b) Predominantly inattentive in which the majority of symptoms (six or more) are in the inattention category, and fewer than six symptoms of hyperactivity-impulsivity are present, although hyperactivity-impulsivity may still be present to some degree; and (c) Combined hyperactive-impulsive and inattentive where six or more symptoms of inattention and six or more symptoms of hyperactivity-impulsivity are present (*DSM-IV-TR*).

Children with the predominantly inattentive subtype of ADHD are less likely to act out or have difficulties getting along with other children. They may sit quietly, but they are not paying attention to what they are doing. Therefore, the child may be overlooked, and parents and teachers may not notice that he or she has ADHD. Most children have the combined type of ADHD.

Etiology

In the past, ADHD has been considered primarily a disorder of childhood, but research has documented cases of this multifactorial disorder across the life span and identified both genetic predisposition and neurobiological deregulation as contributing factors. These etiologic factors lead to a neuropsychological inhibitory deficit that contributes to the specific impairments typical for ADHD at all ages. There is strong evidence for genetic predisposition, including a review of twin studies that demonstrated heritability of up to 76% (Faraone et al., 2005). There is strong evidence for organic brain abnormalities in individuals with ADHD. For example, Castellanos et al. (2002) found based on imaging studies that activity in nearly all brain regions was significantly decreased in children and adolescents with ADHD when compared to normal controls. Interestingly, the presenting characteristics of the disorder tend to become more nonspecific over time, even though the genetics and neurobiology are stable (Schmidt & Petermann, 2009).

ADHD in preschoolers

US and international studies document the prevalence of ADHD in preschoolers as anywhere from 2–6% (e.g. Lavigne et al., 1996; Posner et al., 2007). In this age group, the diagnosis is usually made using rating scales that are completed by parents or caregivers, healthcare providers, and day-care or preschool personnel. Symptoms on rating scales that describe ADHD in preschool children include problems with maintaining attention over time, high levels of distractibility, excessive running or climbing, not complying with instructions, and having difficulty sitting still (DuPaul et al., 1998). It is easy to see why these symptoms would have a negative impact, perhaps throughout his or her lifetime, on a person's quality of life, which underscores the need for early diagnosis and early intervention for children exhibiting these symptoms.

ADHD in school-aged children and adolescents

The prevalence rate of ADHD among school children and adolescents ranges from 3.2% to 15.8%, depending on the classification system used, with rates between 5% and 7% reported most often. In addition, boys are two to four times more likely to be diagnosed with ADHD than girls. As with preschoolers, diagnosis depends on reports of parents, teachers, and educators, but in this age group self-report is added to proxy reports by others (Schmidt & Petermann, 2009). In addition, assessment of attention span in these older children can be assisted by computer-based instruments. Untreated ADHD puts children and adolescents at high risk for negative development in many areas of life, particularly because of the high rate of comorbid disorders such as oppositional behavior (in up to 65% of cases), anxiety disorders (in about 23% of cases), and learning disorders such as dyslexia and dyscalculia (Petty et al., 2009; Souza, Pinheiroi, & Mattos, 2005). Emotional issues are common in older school-age children and increase in frequency during adolescence. These may result, in part, from peer rejection and feeling different from other children. These children and adolescents may develop relationships with other children with similar issues, which may increase functional difficulties and lead to risky behaviors including substance abuse (Bizzarri et al., 2007; Brook et al., 2008).

Psychopharmacologic management of ADHD

According to the National Institutes of Mental Health (2008), treatment focuses on symptom reduction and functional improvement, and may include medication, psychotherapy, psychoeducation, or a combination of these treatment modalities. Stimulants are still the most common class of drugs used for treating ADHD, although there is increasing use of non-stimulants as first-line pharmacologic management. The aim of medication management is to reduce hyperactivity and impulsivity and to improve focus. Coordination may also improve after institution of effective medication management. Often several different medications or dosages must be tried before finding the right combination for any particular child. Careful monitoring in the child's medical home is mandatory. Extended release forms of most stimulants and other non-stimulants are available and may make it unnecessary for a child to take medication at school. A list of common medications used in ADHD management and the approved age for use follows (see Table 3.1). ADHD can be diagnosed and medications prescribed by physicians in all states, and in some states also by clinical psychologists and advanced registered nurse practitioners.

Medication guides for each of these medications are available from the U.S. Food and Drug Administration (FDA).

Table 3.1 ADHD Medications Approved by U.S. Food and Drug Administration (FDA)*

Trade Name	Generic Name	Approved Age
Adderall	amphetamine	3 and older
Adderall XR	amphetamine (extended release)	6 and older
Concerta	methylphenidate (long-acting)	6 and older
Daytrana	methylphenidate patch	6 and older
Desoxyn	methamphetamine hydrochloride	6 and older
Dexedrine	dextroamphetamine	3 and older
Dextrostat	dextroamphetamine	3 and older
Focalin	dexmethylphenidate	6 and older
Focalin XR	dexmethylphenidate (extended release)	6 and older
Metadate ER	methylphenidate (extended release)	6 and older
Metadate CD	methylphenidate (extended release)	6 and older
Methylin	methylphenidate (oral solution and chewable tablets)	6 and older
Ritalin	methylphenidate	6 and older
Ritalin SR	methylphenidate (extended release)	6 and older
Ritalin LA	methylphenidate (long-acting)	6 and older
Strattera	atomoxetine	6 and older
Vyvanse	lisdexamfetamine dimesylate	6 and older

*U.S. Department of Health and Human Services, National Institute of Mental Health. (2008). Attention Deficit Hyperactivity Disorder. NIH Publication No. 08–3672. http://www.nimh .nih.gov/health/publications/attention-deficit-hyperactivity-disorder/adhd_booklet.pdf

The most commonly reported side effects of stimulant medications are decreased appetite, sleep problems, anxiety, and irritability. Some children also report mild stomachaches or headaches. Most side effects are minor and disappear over time or if the dosage level is lowered. A few children develop sudden, repetitive movements or sounds called tics. These tics may or may not be noticeable. Changing the medication dosage may make tics go away. Some children also may have a personality change, such as appearing "flat" or without emotion. In 2007, the FDA required that all makers of ADHD medications develop patient medication guides that contain information about the risks associated with the medications. The guides must alert families that the medications may lead to possible cardiovascular (heart and blood) or psychiatric problems. The agency undertook this precaution when a review of data found that ADHD patients with existing heart conditions had a slightly higher risk of strokes, heart attacks, and/or sudden death when taking the medications. The review also found in patients without a history of psychiatric problems a slight increased risk, about 1 in 1,000, for medication-related psychiatric problems, such as hearing voices, having hallucinations, becoming suspicious for no reason, or becoming manic. The FDA recommends that any treatment plan for ADHD include an initial health history, including family history, and examination for existing cardiovascular and psychiatric problems.

One ADHD medication, the non-stimulant atomoxetine (Strattera), carries another warning. Studies show that children and adolescents who take atomoxetine are more likely to have suicidal thoughts than children and teenagers with ADHD who do not take it (NIMH, 2008).

Psychotherapeutic/behavioral management of ADHD (NIMH, 2008)

Different types of psychotherapy and psychoeducation are used for ADHD. Behavioral therapy aims to help a child change his or her behavior. It might involve practical assistance, such as help organizing tasks or completing schoolwork, or working through emotionally difficult events. Behavioral therapy also teaches a child how to monitor his or her own behavior. Learning to give oneself praise or rewards for acting in a desired way, such as controlling anger or thinking before acting, is another goal of behavioral therapy. It is important that children learn social skills, such as how to wait their turn, share toys, ask for help, or respond to teasing. Learning to read facial expressions and the tone of voice in others, and learning how to respond appropriately, can also be part of social skills training. Sometimes, the whole family may need therapy. Therapists can help family members find better ways to handle disruptive behaviors and to encourage behavior changes.

Application to nursing and multidisciplinary practice

Caring for a child with ADHD requires a team approach with the family at the center of the team. Nursing and other disciplines can offer suggestions to children and families that might reduce the negative impact on children and family quality of life. For example, parenting skills training helps parents learn how to use a system of rewards and consequences to change a child's behavior. Parents are taught to give immediate and positive feedback for behaviors they want to encourage, and ignore or redirect behaviors they want to discourage. In some cases, the use of "time-outs" may be used when the child's behavior gets out of control. In a time-out, the child is removed from the upsetting situation and sits alone for a short time to calm down. Parents are also encouraged to share a pleasant or relaxing activity with the child, to notice and point out what the child does well, and to praise the child's strengths and abilities. They may also learn to structure situations in more positive ways. For example, they may restrict the number of playmates to one or two, so that their child does not become overstimulated. Or, if the child has trouble completing tasks, parents can help their child divide large tasks into smaller, more manageable steps. Also, parents may benefit from learning stress-management techniques to increase their own ability to deal with frustration so that they can respond calmly to their child's behavior. Finally, support groups help parents and families connect with others who have similar problems and concerns. Groups often meet regularly to share frustrations and successes, to exchange information about recommended specialists and strategies, and to talk with experts.

THE CHILD WITH INTELLECTUAL DISABILITY

Definition and presenting signs and symptoms

According to the Centers for Disease Control and Prevention (Parker et al., 2010), intellectual disability is characterized both by significantly subaverage scores on tests of cognitive ability or intelligence and by limitations in the ability to function in areas of daily life such as communication, self-care, and getting along in social situations and school activities. Intellectual disability is sometimes referred to as cognitive disability or mental retardation. By definition, intellectual disability begins before a child reaches the age of 18 years.

Prevalence of intellectual disability

Intellectual disability is the most common developmental disability in children. Prevalence studies supported by the CDC (Metropolitan Atlanta

COMMON DEVELOPMENTAL/
LEARNING DISABILITIES

Developmental Disabilities Surveillance Program) documented rates of intellectual disabilities (score of 70 or below on IQ test) of between 12 and 16 per 1,000 school-aged children (Karapurkar et al., 1996/2000), although other studies (e.g., Battaglia & Carey, 2003) put the prevalence rates much higher, at 1–10% of the US population. In 2006, nearly 614,000 children ages 3 to 21 in the United States had some level of intellectual disability and needed special education in school (U.S. Department of Education, 2006).

Etiology

For many children, the cause of their intellectual disability is not known (Parker et al., 2010), although causes can be roughly categorized as resulting from genetic problems, problems during the prenatal period such as ingestion of toxic substances or infection, perinatal problems, or childhood injury or disease. In fact, mental retardation (MR) is one of the few clinically important disorders for which the etiology and pathogenesis is still poorly understood (Battaglia & Carey, 2003). It is a condition of great concern for public health and society, and recent advances in genetic knowledge offer hope for earlier, more accurate diagnosis. Some of the most common known causes of congenital intellectual disability are Down syndrome, infections such as cytomegalovirus, and perinatal asphyxia. Acquired causes of intellectual disability include, among others, serious head injury, stroke, or infections such as meningitis or encephalitis.

Diagnosis

Intellectual functioning, or IQ, is usually measured by an IQ test with an average score of 100. People scoring below 70 to 75 are thought to have an intellectual disability. To measure adaptive behavior, professionals look at what a child can do in comparison to other children of his or her age. Certain skills are important to adaptive behavior, including daily living, language, and social skills. Cytogenetic studies and neuro-imaging can identify some common causes of intellectual disability, such as Down syndrome (Battaglia & Carey, 2003). Although there are no specific phenotypic characteristics that are associated with all types of intellectual disability, many children with these disorders have evidence of microcephaly (head circumference below the 5th percentile for age).

Children with intellectual disability can and do learn new skills, but they develop more slowly than children with average intelligence and adaptive skills. There are different degrees of intellectual disability, ranging from mild to profound. A person's level of intellectual disability can be defined, in part, by his or her developmental or intelligence quotient but the types and amount of support the person needs is often more diagnostic than a number. Even within a particular diagnosis, such as Down syndrome, there is a wide range of intellectual and adaptive capabilities.

DOWN SYNDROME AS EXEMPLAR OF INTELLECTUAL DISABILITY

Down syndrome (trisomy 21) is the result of an extra copy of all or part of chromosome 21, the smallest chromosome in humans. It is likely that the small number of genes on this chromosome contributes to its lack of lethality and thus its stability in the human gene pool (Einfeld & Brown, 2010). Down syndrome (DS) was identified as a distinct condition in the late 19th century, and was originally called "mongolism" because of apparent facial resemblance to Asian races. Advances in genetics demonstrated that DS could be caused by trisomy of only part of chromosome 21 and led to the identification of the distal long arm of the chromosome as the "sensitive" region of chromosome 21 responsible for the DS attributes. Currently, DS is estimated to occur in 1.4 per 1000 live births (Centers for Disease Control, 2006).

The standard for screening for DS prenatally is by blood test followed by ultrasound, and definitive diagnosis is achieved through amniocentesis or chorionic villus sampling, which carry a 1% increased risk of miscarriage. In addition, there is often a two- to three-week delay before cells are cultured and results are available to the pregnant woman. Early studies of a blood test that scans DNA from the small number of fetal cells in maternal blood and identifies those that show aneuploidy (extra copies of chromosomes) have been effective in diagnosing DS noninvasively; the test can be done at 12 weeks of gestation, and provides results in a couple of days. If larger studies validate the test, it will be the first diagnostic noninvasive test for DS (Fan et al., 2008). Children born with DS characteristics undergo genetic testing soon after birth.

Characteristics common to individuals with DS include some degree of intellectual impairment, marked flattening of the back of the skull, a slight slant to the eyelids, additional skin folds at the inner aspects of the eye, depressed nasal bridge, small ears, small mouth, hypotonia of major muscle groups, small hands and feet, and ligamentous laxity (Hayes, 2007). Some children with DS have only a few of these characteristics, while some have most of them. The degree of intellectual disability ranges widely in individuals with DS. Alzheimer-like dementia is found in almost all individuals with DS who are older than 40 years, and DS is known to be associated with a high incidence of leukemia (Einfeld & Brown, 2010) and other medical conditions such as cardiac disorders, hearing loss, and vision loss.

There is new hope for medical management of this ancient disorder. Cutting edge research into the pathogenic mechanisms of trisomy 21 has the potential of identifying ways to regulate the function of the genes on chromosome 21 responsible for the DS phenotype, and thus improve brain function in individuals born with DS (Einfeld & Brown, 2010).

Application to clinical practice

Although children born with Down syndrome are now living longer, they may experience compromised musculoskeletal and neurologic function over time, especially instability of the cervical spine, hips, and knees that may negatively impact their function and quality of life. Healthcare providers evaluating children with Down syndrome must be alert to these disorders and must understand that radiographs of children with Down syndrome are sometimes difficult to interpret and are not comparable to radiographs of children without Down syndrome (Pizzutillo & Herman, 2006). Research evidence shows that early, intensive medical and educational intervention has a significant positive influence on the child's development as well as his or her integration into the community (Feeley & Jones, 2008).

THE CHILD WITH AN AUTISM SPECTRUM DISORDER

Definition and presenting signs and symptoms

Most individuals with autism demonstrate symptoms including deficits in reciprocal social interaction, communication, and language, and by stereotyped and repetitive interests and behaviors (Johnson, 2004). Autism is in the category of pervasive developmental disorder (PDD) according to the *DSM-IV-TR* (American Psychiatric Association, 2000). Two other PDDs, Asperger syndrome and PDD-not otherwise specified are also on the autism spectrum. Together, these disorders are generally referred to as autism spectrum disorders (ASDs). All of these disorders have some similar characteristics but age of onset and symptom severity differ widely among individuals with autism spectrum disorders.

Prevalence of ASDs

It is estimated that between 1 in 80 and 1 in 240 with an average of 1 in 110 children in the United States have an ASD, and similar rates have been identified in Asia and in Europe (Centers for Disease Control and Prevention, 2007). Autism occurs in all racial, ethnic, and socioeconomic groups, but is four to five times more common in boys than in girls. Risk factors for autism include having a twin with autism; having a sibling with autism; or having an identifiable genetic, neurologic, or metabolic disorder such as fragile X or Down syndrome.

Diagnosis

The median age of earliest ASD diagnosis is between 4.5 and 5.5 years, but for 51–91 percent of children with an ASD, developmental concerns were raised before the age of three years (CDC, 2007). Recent studies indicate that a diagnosis of autism at age 2 can be reliable, valid, and stable (NIH/NCBDDD, 2008). The *DSM-IV-TR* provides standardized criteria to help diagnose ASD. In addition, there are a number of diagnostic scales designed to capture the deficits and aberrant behaviors characteristic of autism, including the Autism Diagnostic Interview-Revised (ADI-R) (Lord et al., 1997) and the Autism Diagnostic Observation Schedule (ADOS)(Lord et al.). The ADI-R is a 93-item questionnaire administered in an interview with parents; it measures social interaction, communication, and the presence of restricted, repetitive and stereotyped behaviors. The diagnostic algorithms focus on behaviors and skills that were ever present as well as on current behaviors and skills, taking into account age of symptom onset. The ADOS is a semi-structured instrument designed to evaluate children based on behaviors common to children with autism and also on the absence or aberancy of behaviors and skills that are normally present in children of the age of the presenting child.

Recently, the American Academy of Neurology and the Child Neurology Society published a series of guidelines for developmental surveillance and screening for autism spectrum disorders (available at http://www.guideline.gov) that recommend routine developmental surveillance at least through school age if any concerns are raised about social acceptance, learning, or behavior. Recommended screening tools include the Ages and Stages Questionnaire, the BRIGANCE Screens, the Child Development Inventories, and the Parents' Evaluations of Developmental Status, with further diagnosis using the Checklist for Autism in Toddlers (CHAT) or the Autism Screening Questionnaire, in which missing developmental milestones that show sensitivity to autism are outlined. In addition, there are recommendations for careful monitoring of siblings of children with autism and for laboratory evaluations, including audiologic assessment and lead screening for any child showing signs of developmental delay and/or autism. Links to downloadable screening tools for general development and ASDs are provided on the guideline.gov web site under "autism."

Until recently, children with high-functioning autism or Asperger syndrome were often missed on screening. However, there are now several tools, including the Autism Spectrum Screening Questionnaire, that can reliably screen for social and behavioral impairments in children who do not show the significant language delays common in children with more severe presentations of autism (CDC, 2007).

Application to clinical practice

Ideally, management of the child with autism, like children with a variety of other chronic health conditions, is a team affair, with a variety of clinical and educational disciplines working with the family who heads the team (Eddy & Engel, 2008). Treatment for children with ASDs has to be individualized. Some children respond better to one type of treatment than to another, and healthcare providers need to listen to family wishes regarding treatment and to talk with the family about risks and benefits of potential interventions. Most efficacious treatments for autism include well-planned, structured teaching of specific skills (CDC, 2007). As with other disabilities of early childhood, early intervention services can greatly improve a child's development.

Healthcare providers need to include regular medical and dental screenings in the management plan for children with ASDs, as they get sick or injured like all children. The child's team must also pay attention to the child's mental health, as new behavioral issues may be related to the ASD but might also be new presentations of a separate mental or physical health condition. The National Institutes of Health/National Center on Birth Defects and Developmental Disabilities provides a comprehensive webpage for healthcare providers about caring for children with ASDs at http://www.cdc.gov/ncbddd/autism/hcp.html.

MIA – A CHILD WITH DOWN SYNDROME

Remember Mia, our 5-year-old girl with Down syndrome whom we met in the introductory chapter? Now that we have discussed developmental and learning disabilities at length, there are important health and developmental differences that the clinician needs to attend to in caring for Mia. Recall that Mia came to the clinic with acute otitis media. Although primary care providers might choose to watch and wait rather than treat otitis media in a healthy 5-year-old with a normal immune system, there are diagnosis-related issues that might require a different choice for Mia. The shorter, broader Eustachian tubes common in individuals with Down syndrome make reflux of fluid to the middle ear and accompanying acute bacterial otitis media more likely. In addition, children with Down syndrome often have compromised immune systems that do not allow them to localize infections easily. Bacteria from the middle ear has the potential to spread to the brain and even to result in widespread sepsis. Therefore, Mia is likely to require antibiotic therapy where a non-Downs child might not. Mia's care team needs to monitor resolution of her otitis and continue careful surveillance for the other health issues common to individuals with Down syndrome, including cardiac abnormalities; acute leukemias; and instability of cervical spine, knee, and hip joints. A clinic visit for an acute problem might also provide an opportunity to talk with family members and other healthcare and educational team members about Mia's future.

REFERENCES

American Psychiatric Association. (2000). *Diagnostic and statistical manual of mental disorders* (4th ed., text rev.). DSM-IV-TR workgroup. Washington, DC: American Psychiatric Association.

Battaglia, A., & Carey, J.C. (2003). Diagnostic evaluation of developmental delay/mental retardation: An overview. *American Journal of Medical Genetics Part C: Seminars in Medical Genetics, 117C*, 3–14. doi: 10.1002/ajmg.c.10015

Bizzarri, J.V., Rucci, P., Sbrana, A., et al. (2007). Reasons for substance use and vulnerability factors in patients with substance use disorder and anxiety or mood disorders. *Addict Behaviors, 32*, 384–391. doi: 10.1016/j.addbeh.2006.04.005.

Brook, J.S., Duan, T., Zhang, C., et al. (2008). The association between Attention Deficit Hyperactivity Disorder in adolescence and smoking in adulthood. *American Journal of Addictions, 17*, 54–59. doi: 10.1080/10550490701756039.

Castellanos, F.X., Lee, P.P., Sharp, W., et al. (2002). Developmental trajectories of brain volume abnormalities in children and adolescents with attention-deficit/hyperactivity disorder. *JAMA, 288*, 1740–1748. doi: 10.1001/jama.288.14.1740.

Centers for Disease Control and Prevention. (2006). Improved national prevalence estimates for 18 selected major birth defects – United States, 1999–2001. *MMWR. Morbidity and Mortality Weekly Report, 54*, 1301–1305.

Centers for Disease Control and Prevention. (2007). Prevalence of autism spectrum disorders–autism and developmental disabilities monitoring network, 14 sites, United States, 2002. *MMWR. Surveillance Summaries: Morbidity and Mortality Weekly Report 56*, 12–28.

DuPaul, G.J., Anastopoulus, A.D., Power, T.J., et al. (1998). Parent ratings of Attention-Deficit/Hyperactivity-Disorder: Factor structure, normative data and psychometric properties. *Journal of Psychopathology and Behavioral Assessment, 20*, 83–102. doi: 10.1023/A:1023087410712.

Eddy, L., & Engel, J. (2008). The impact of child disability type on the family. *Rehabilitation Nursing, 33*(3), 98–103.

Einfeld, S.J., & Brown, R. (2010). Down syndrome – new prospects for an ancient disorder. *JAMA, 303*, 2525–2526.

Fan, H.C., Blumenfeld, Y.J., Chitkara, U., et al. (2008). Noninvasive diagnosis of fetal aneuploidy by shotgun sequencing DNA from maternal blood. *Proceedings of the National Academy of Science USA, 105*(42), 16266–16271.

Faraone, S.V., Perlis, R.H., Doyle, A.E., et al. (2005). Molecular genetics of attention-deficit/hyperactivity disorder. *Biological Psychiatry, 57*, 1313–1323. doi: 10.1016/j.biopsych.2004.11.024.

COMMON DEVELOPMENTAL/
LEARNING DISABILITIES

Feeley, K., & Jones, E. (2008). Down's syndrome, research and practice. *Journal of the Sarah Duffen Centre/University Of Portsmouth, 12*(2), 153–163.

Hayes, C. (2007). Down syndrome: Caring holistically in primary health care. *British Journal of Community Nursing, 12*(9), 404–406.

Johnson, C.P. (2004). Early clinical characteristics of children with autism. In V.B. Gupta, V.B. (Ed.), *Autistic spectrum disorders in children* (pp. 85–123). New York, NY: Marcel Dekker.

Karapurkar Bhasin, T., Brocksen, S., Avchen, R.N., et al. (1996/2000). Prevalence of four developmental disabilities among children aged 8 years. *MMWR Surveillance Summaries, 55*(SS01):1–9.

Lavigne, J.V., Gibbons, R.D., Christoffel, K.K., et al. (1996). Prevalence rates and correlates of psychiatric disorders among preschool children. *Journal of American Academy of Child & Adolescent Psychiatry, 35*, 204–214. doi: 10.1097/00004583-199602000-00014.

Lord, C., Pickles, A., Mclennan, J., et al. (1997). Diagnosing autism: Analyses of data from the Autism Diagnostic Interview. *Journal of Autism and Developmental Disorders, 27*, 501–517.

National Institute of Mental Health. (2008). *Attention deficit hyperactivity disorder* (NIH Publication No. 08-3572). Retrieved from http://www.nimh.nih.gov/health/publications/attention-deficit-hyperactivity-disorder/adhd_booklet.pdf

Parker, S.E., Mai, C.T., Canfield, M.A., et al. (2010). National Birth Defects Prevention Network. *BirthDefects Research* (Part A), *88*, 1008–1016.

Petty, C.R., Monuteaux, M.C., Mick, E., et al. (2009). Parsing the familiality of oppositional defiant disorder from that of conduct disorder: A familial risk analysis. *Journal of Psychiatric Reserch, 43*, 345–352. doi: 10.1016/j.jpsychires.2008.03.010.

Posner, K., Melvin, G.A., Murray, D.W., et al. (2007). Clinical presentation of attention-deficit/hyperactivity disorder in preschool children: The preschoolers with attention-deficit/hyperactivity disorder treatment Study (PATS). *Journal of Child & Adolescent Psychopharmacology, 17*, 547–562. doi: 10.1089/cap.2007.0075

Pizzutillo, P.D., & Herman, M.J. (2006). Cervical spine management in children with Down syndrome. *Current Opinion in Orthopedics, 17*(3), 260–263.

Schmidt, S., & Petermann, F. (2009). Developmental psychopathology: Attention deficit hyperactivity disorder (ADHD). *BMC Psychiatry, 9*(58). doi: 10.1186/147-244X-9-58.

Souza, I., Pinheiroi, M.A., & Mattos, P. (2005). Anxiety disorders in an attention-deficit/hyperactivity disorder clinical sample. *Arqu Neuropsiquiatr, 63*, 407–409.

U.S. Department of Education. (2006). Office of Special Educaton and Rehabilitative Services, Office of Special Education Programs. *26th annual (2004) report to Congress on the implementation of the Individuals with Disabilities Education Act*, Vol. 1. Washington, DC: Author.

COMMON DEVELOPMENTAL/
LEARNING DISABILITIES

CHAPTER 4
CARING FOR CHILDREN WITH FEEDING AND COMMUNICATION DIFFERENCES

Lisa Lyons

Caring for Children with Special Healthcare Needs and Their Families: A Handbook for Healthcare Professionals, First Edition. Edited by Linda L. Eddy.
© 2013 John Wiley & Sons, Inc. Published 2013 by John Wiley & Sons, Inc.

In the fourth edition of the highly popular *What to Expect When You're Expecting* (2008), authors Murkoff and Mazel provide a pregnancy guide that "reassuringly answers the questions of mothers- and fathers-to-be, from the planning stage through postpartum." It would be helpful for a similar guide to be available to parents and care providers of infants and young children in terms of expectations for early feeding and communication skills. When a child is unable to eat easily for proper weight gain and hydration, or in an accepted, safe manner free from aspiration or choking risk, it can be extremely stressful to a new parent. If feeding or drinking skills do not advance in an anticipated way in terms of cultural expectations, it can be confusing and concerning. Early feeding skills are considered a basic life function.

The development of effective communications skills is expected also to naturally occur. If a child is unable to hear, to understand, to speak, or to interact in ways that are expected for "one's age," anxiety can occur for parents. Early feeding and/or communication impairments may be the first signals that a child has special healthcare needs.

As Shipley and McAfee (2009) highlight, during initial and subsequent visits with pediatric patients, it is helpful to:

- Identify the child's medical status

- Identify the child's feeding and communicative status

- Be aware of dietary restrictions

- Be aware of communication status

- Converse with caregivers as to their questions or concerns regarding feeding or communicative status.

This chapter will provide a basic guide as to "What to Expect" for infants through early school-age children concerning common feeding and communication milestones. Given the complexity of feeding and communication milestones, no list can be all-inclusive. The primary care provider reader will be cued to what to be on the look out for to best determine if further assessment and/or remediation is needed. After review of typical milestones, common early feeding difficulties and management strategies will be discussed. Similarly, common speech and language delays or impairments will be presented. The chapter concludes with a description of then professions of speech-language pathology and audiology and when to refer someone to those professionals, and highlights common treatment strategies for the early communicative disorders outlined.

OVERVIEW OF EARLY FEEDING SKILLS

When a baby is first born, he or she is expected to be able to engage in oral intake via sucking at the breast or bottle that is safe, efficient, and positively tolerated. "Safe" refers to the ability to take in food or fluid in a manner that progresses from mouth to stomach without risk of it being aspirated (going into the airway tube rather than esophagus to stomach) or becoming an airway obstruction. "Efficiency" refers to the ability to take in food or fluids in a manner that calorie and hydration goals are met without undue calorie burn. "Positively tolerated" refers to intake of food or drink in a manner that an infant or child engages in without dislike or discomfort.

Children with special healthcare needs may not be able to eat enough, may not be able to eat safely, or may exhibit growth retardation despite adequate caloric intake. "Feeding problems can be defined objectively by a child's growth chart. Poor growth will first be reflected in weight, then length, and finally head circumference" (Blackman, 1990). In cases of typical early feeding and drinking skills, there is a developmental progression as babies mature. The developmental milestones are presented in chronological outline below. "When evaluating a child who was born prematurely, it is important to consider the child's adjusted age rather than chronological age" (Shipley & McAfee, 2009).

Developmental feeding milestones: Gestational period through age 7

- Nonnutritive suck reflex present at 11 weeks gestation

- Rooting reflex present at 32 weeks gestation

- Suck-swallow reflex of sufficient strength and coordination for oral feeding to begin at 34–35 weeks gestation

- From approximately 34 weeks gestation for nearly first year of life, baby receives all nourishment, if able, through nipple feedings of breast milk and/or formula.

- Readiness for exposure to early spoon feedings by evidence of: sufficient head and trunk control for supportive seating, lip closure around spoon, decrease of tongue thrust, and ability to strip smooth small volume of puree from spoon. This is typically around 6 to 9 months chronological age. During this period, primary nourishment remains via nipple feeds as early spoon feedings advance.

- Infant develops cues for feeding, uses facial expression to convey likes and dislikes, and ideally, mealtimes become predictable and linked to family schedule.

- At approximately 7 months through 9 months, unsupported seating advances as does ability to hold items independently.

- Assisted cup drinking may be introduced as may early quick-to-dissolve early finger foods. A "bite" is what is utilized to break a piece of food off and introduce into mouth, whereas "chewing" refers to breaking up of the piece within the mouth. Due to immature hand control and safety awareness, infants in this stage are at particular choking risk if they introduce food or nonfood items into the mouth that cannot or should not be appropriately masticated and swallowed.

- By 9 months, increased desire to "self-feed" emerges. There may be impatience if caregiver is slow in presenting in food.

- During 10 to 12 months as teeth erupt, tongue lateralization for chewing advances, and jaw and tongue work independently, early "eating" skills advance. Cup drinking increases and nipple feedings decrease.

- During 13 to 18 months, chewing transitions from munch "up and down" tongue pattern to rotary pattern. The strength and coordination of the tongue, however, is not fully mature, which is why toddlers and young children gravitate toward "processed foods" that are easy to masticate and swallow.

- Straw drinking may be introduced, and unlidded cup drinking becomes easier during this 13- to 18-month phase. Nipple feeding is replaced by cup drinking typically during this phase.

- As children progress from age 1 1/2 years to their second birthday, teeth eruption continues. With sufficient tongue and swallow coordination, they can begin to be exposed to "mixed textures" such as cereal with milk or soup with particles.

- By the second birthday, the child feeds self most of the time and is effectively utilizing child-safe utensils.

- By the third birthday, all 20 deciduous teeth are present. Coordination for chewing and swallowing advances allowing for greater variation in food textures, with diet more closing matching that of the family's by fourth birthday.

- Between fourth and seventh year, coordination for chewing and swallowing continues to advance. It is common for child to have strong food likes and dislikes. Deciduous teeth by the seventh year begin to fall out, and during the stage of "loose" or unerupted permanent teeth, feeding skills may be impacted.

OVERVIEW OF EARLY COMMUNICATION SKILLS

The above overview focused on early feeding and drinking skill milestones. "Many of the muscles used for speech production are also used for chewing and swallowing" (Shipley & McAfee, 2009). For this reason, many infants and children who have early feeding challenges also experience early communication challenges. There are helpful resources for parents that will let them know what to expect in terms of early communication milestones. The American Speech Language Hearing Association provides free handouts on a variety of topics through http://www.asha.org. For example, they provide an educational DVD, *Speech, Language, and Hearing Milestones Birth to Age Five*, that primary care practitioners may find helpful to have on hand. The text *Childhood Speech, Language, and Listening Problems: What Every Parent Should Know* by Patricia McAleer Hamaguchi (2001) provides a written resource on early development and common communicative challenges that exist.

The following section provides an overview of developmental milestones of "what to expect" in terms of early communication skills. As with early eating and drinking skills sequences described, description of common milestones from infancy to age 7 is a "general guide" as infants and children develop at different rates.

Developmental communication milestones infancy through age 7

- Birth to 3 months: reacts to sudden noises by crying or body jerk; reacts to familiar people or objects; emerging differential cry for hunger versus pain; watches objects intently; "cooing" early prolonged varied vowel production begins

- 3 months to 6 months: "babbling" early consonant+vowel production with intonation changes; laughs, squeals, turns head to source of sound; uses louder crying or laughing

- 6 to 9 months: begins to comprehend single words; varied intonation of babbling with production of 2+ syllables and varied consonants (m,p,b,d,w);

understands and reacts to facial expression; attempts gestures to early social games or communication such as "bye bye" or "peek-a-boo"; and shakes head to show "no."

- 9 months to 12 months: enjoys sound and action imitation; may show emerging use of "first word approximations" such as "mama" or "dada"; responds to music and voice; begins to understand single requests such as "give it to me"; increasingly uses gestures, cries, or early word attempts to request something; looks at source of sound immediately.

- 12 months to 18 months: growing understanding of vocabulary words with understanding of approximately 50 to 75 words; growing use of word approximations from 3 to 20+ words; points to known people or objects when named; points to simple body parts; increased use of "jargon," which is connected babbling that matches intonation of speech patterns, follows simple one-step commands, and imitates words heard.

- 18 months to 2 years: comprehends approximately 300 hundred words; word use grows, as word approximations are at the 50+ level then early 2-word utterances begin to emerge but there is often decreased speech intelligibility and long pauses between words; speaks often with real words coupled with jargon; often enjoys hearing same story repeated; often expresses strong emotion with cries rather than available words; emerging use of rising intonation to reflect question; begins to use verbs and adjectives; will tell his or her name when asked.

- 2 years to 3 years: understands approximately 900 words; expressive "spoken" vocabulary increases to approximately 500 words with increased use of 3+ and longer word utterances; speech is approximately 50 to 70% intelligible; expresses frustration using words more than cries; emerging eye contact during conversation; greater identification of people and things; improving comprehension of prepositions "in," "on," and "under"; begins to ask "yes/no" questions; increasing "self-talk" during play; early disfluency common with repetition of whole words when excited or mad.

- 3 years to 4 years: understands approximately 1,200 words and utilizes approximately 800 words; asks many "what" and "who" questions; understands simple time concepts, positional words, and simple plot in children's stories; increased use of grammatical markers such as contractions, plurals, and "s"' to mark present tense such as "plays"; word repetition is less frequent and speech is understandable approximately 70 to 80% of the time; can sit and engage in activity for 10 to 15 minutes, initiate conversations; asks questions, sometimes same one repeatedly, and will make comments or observations on activity occurring in environment.

- 4 to 5 years: comprehends 2,500 to 2,800 words and uses up to 2,000; uses pronouns correctly; speaks in complex sentences run together with speech intelligibility at approximately 90% of the time; advanced use of grammatical concepts including past, present, and future regular and irregular verb tense; follows 3-step+ commands; understands common opposites; can describe pictures, make up stories, explain events, play dramatically, listen, and attend to stories and movies longer with increasing time duration.

- 5 years to 7 years: advancing improvements in pronunciation, sentence structure, word use, attention span, listening, and memory.

The above list highlights the common milestones observed in speech, language, and listening. Earliest developing sounds are vowels followed by consonants, but not all consonant production is achieved at once. The ability to produce sounds is impacted by hearing and stage of development of articulators such as teeth, tongue, lips, and palate. A variety of speech sound developmental charts are available that demonstrate the particular age when speech sounds are acquired. In addition to speech sound production, factors that affect communication include voice, fluency, and nasal resonance.

SCREENING OF EARLY FEEDING AND COMMUNICATION SKILLS

The above guidelines for early feeding and communication development highlight the complexity of such development. When meeting with a caregiver of an infant and young child, it is helpful to ask if that person has concerns about the infant or child's skills and for the primary healthcare provider him or herself to be on the lookout as caregivers are not always cognizant of delays or impairments when they exist. Often a parent's intuition is right and if concerned, referral to a specialist can be helpful to explore feeding and/or communication skills.

Impaired feeding skills

In regard to early nutrition and growth, the primary healthcare provider reader is referred to an excellent resource, the "Nutrition and Growth" chapter in *The Physician's Guide to Caring for Children with Disabilities and Chronic Conditions* (2000), which describes prevalence, etiology for failure to thrive, diagnosis and evaluation, and management of oral motor and behavioral feeding disorders. Children with special healthcare needs are at risk for developing problems with nutrition and growth. Blackman (1990) in his chapter "Feeding Problems" in *Medical Aspects of Developmental Disabilities in Children*

Birth to Three summarizes challenges that place infants and young children at particular risk for insufficient caloric intake:

- central nervous system immaturity

- central nervous system damage

- chromosomal abnormalities

- cardiac or respiratory disease

- kidney disease

- structural abnormalities such as craniofacial conditions, including cleft palate

- mechanical problems such as gastroesophageal reflux, delayed gastric emptying

- significant developmental delay

- behavioral or sensory difficulties

- impaired parent-child interaction

Oral and/or pharyngeal dysphagia may affect a child's ability to safely ingest sufficient calories or to advance in age-appropriate feeding or drinking skills. Other issues, either in isolation or co-existing, may be present that can impact early feeding skills, such as gastroesophageal reflux, acute or chronic disorders, prematurity, and high metabolic demands. In addition to monitoring of weight, length, weight-to-length ratio, and head circumference, primary care providers may need to take a feeding history, including a 24-hour history of dietary intake; directly observe feedings; evaluate and diagnose failure to thrive and/or gastroesophageal reflux; screen for oral motor dysfunction and/or behavioral issues related to feedings; and refer the child for comprehensive evaluation by feeding specialists (Jepsen & Nickel, 2000).

If there is concern with aspiration risk, breast or bottle intake, or failure to advance in drinking or feeding skills, a referral to a feeding specialist is recommended. Particular risk factors include: impaired lip closure, drooling or impaired saliva or food/drink control, impaired sucking, tonic biting, delayed chewing skills, tongue thrusting, limited food textures for age, sensory defensiveness, coughing or gagging with feeding, history of dehydration, impaired weight gain, and/or aspiration pneumonias.

CARING FOR CHILDREN WITH FEEDING AND COMMUNICATION DIFFERENCES

If medical evaluation confirms concern with any of the above, further evaluation for etiology of failure to thrive, gastroesophageal reflux (GER), and/or aspiration is required. In turn, management of oral motor and behavioral feeding disorder, oral motor dysfunction, and GER can occur, but there may be need for hospitalization, medication, non-oral feeds, and/or surgical interventions. Safety and maintenance of hydration and nutritional needs is critical, yet this should be coupled with an awareness of the long-term goal of optimizing the potential for safe, efficient, positively tolerated oral feedings across development stages. A team approach is often most effective in management and may involve the specialists of pediatrics, gastroenterology, nutrition, speech/language pathology, nursing, and/or occupational therapy.

Impaired communication skills

There are numerous conditions, congenital and acquired, that can impact communication skills throughout all stages of life. Traumatic injuries to the face and oral musculature from motor vehicle accidents or other blunt force trauma can result in impaired communication. Sometimes more subtle occurrences such as anoxia during the birth process can result in brain impairments that are not originally appreciated at the time of birth.

In "Craniofacial Disorders" in *The Physician's Guide to Caring for Children with Disabilities and Chronic Conditions,* Letcher-Glembo (2000) reviews anatomy, physiology, and clinical problems commonly associated with cleft and other craniofacial conditions. Craniofacial anomalies range from simple (e.g., cleft lip) to complex (e.g., Treacher Collins syndrome) and may be isolated or associated with other congenital defects, increasing the risk of special needs in communication. Children with craniofacial anomalies are at increased risk of not only early feeding challenges but for permanent or fluctuating hearing loss, higher incidence of middle-ear disease (Volk, Arnold, & Brodsky, 1992), and dentoskeletal differences (Roba & Bochacki, 1992), any of which can impact early communication.

Children with craniofacial anomalies should be evaluated fully within the first few days after birth or at the latest within the first few weeks of life (ACPA, 1993). Ongoing evaluations are required because of the complex and longitudinal nature of difficulties associated with craniofacial anomalies. "The primary health care provider can promote optimal care by prompt identification and referral of the infant and family to a craniofacial disorders team" (Letcher-Glembo, 2000). The following, as outlined by Letcher-Glembo, are the responsibilities of the primary healthcare provider in the initial evaluation of infants with craniofacial anomalies:

- Perform an evaluation for minor physical anomalies to determine need for further evaluation (e.g., blood chromosomal analysis) and referral to a medical geneticist to assist with the diagnosis of a birth defect syndrome and for counseling regarding risk of recurrence.

- Evaluate the infant for other associated defects such as cervical spine anomaly or congenital heart defect.

- Identify newborns and children with feeding and/or swallowing difficulties who are at risk for weight loss, malnutrition, and/or dehydration, and make a referral as needed to professionals with expertise in feeding children.

- Refer the child and family to cleft/craniofacial disorders team.

- Provide advocacy, information, and ongoing support to the family in conjunction with the craniofacial team.

Other conditions are not as obvious as a cleft or other craniofacial condition. At times it takes the parent or insight of the primary care provider to observe that an infant or young child is falling behind or is different from their chronological peers in early communication development. If the primary healthcare provider or the parent has questions, it can be helpful to seek the professional opinion of a speech/language pathologist. It is not wise to assume the child will outgrow the problem, and early intervention can help to alleviate the problem before it worsens or impacts other areas of function.

A "communicative disorder is a perceived deviation from normal hearing, speech, or language that interferes with communication, or calls adverse attention to the person possessing it, or causes him or her to be self-conscious or maladjusted" (Silverman, 1995). The first part of his definition highlights the importance of "normal hearing." Adequate hearing and middle ear function are critical in early communicative development. Inquiring as to whether the infant hearing screening was passed, appropriate follow-up as needed was performed, and obtainment of current otologic status is of importance for primary healthcare providers. Most disorders of hearing are caused by structural deviation or damage to outer, middle, or inner ear, on one or both sides, or to some part of the central auditory nervous system in which the parts of the brain process information inputted by the ears. The amount of difficulty an infant or young child will experience in early communicative development can be impacted by the location and extent of damage to the hearing system.

Beyond the importance of hearing, Silverman outlines primary types of "speech" communicative disorders. Figure 4.1 summarizes communicative disorders described facts and prevalence rate.

To provide further insight, types of speech disorders are described as either disorders of articulation, disorders of fluency, or disorders of receptive or expressive language. *Disorders of articulation* involve errors in one or more

CARING FOR CHILDREN WITH
FEEDING AND COMMUNICATION
DIFFERENCES

- **Articulation Disorders – impairment of the ability to articulate speech sounds.**

  ➤ **The prevalence of speech sound disorders in young children is 8-9%. By the first grade, approximately 5% of children have noticeable speech disorders.**

- **Fluency Disorders – interruption in the flow of speaking characterized by atypical rate, rhythm and repetitions in sounds, syllables, words and phrases. This may be accompanied by excessive tension, struggle behavior and secondary characteristics.**

  ➤ **The prevalence of fluency disorders in young children is 4-5%. The incidence is highest for children between the ages of 2 and 4 years.**

- **Voice Disorders – abnormal production of vocal quality, pitch, loudness and resonance compared to an individual's age and/or sex.**

  ➤ **The prevalence of voice disorders in school-aged children is 6 to 23% with the majority demonstrating hoarseness. The most common cause of hoarseness is vocal nodules.**

- **Phonological Disorders – abnormal development of the sound system of a language and the rules that govern sound combinations. This results in difficulty producing age expected speech sounds.**

  ➤ **The prevalence of phonological disorders in children is 8 to 9%.**

- **Language Disorders – impaired comprehension and/or use of spoken and written language. The disorder may include difficulty with:**
  - **Semantics - meaning of language**
  - **Syntax - grammatical construction of languages**
  - **Pragmatics - social use of language, includes conversational skills**
  - **Phonological Awareness – knowledge of the sound structure of language**
  - **Reading, Spelling and Writing**

  ➤ **The prevalence of language disorders in preschool children is between 6-8%.**
  ➤ **The prevalence of language disorders in early school-age children is between 2 to 8%.**
  ➤ **The prevalence of reading disorders in school-age children is 17%.**

- **Apraxia – Difficulty in initiating and executing the movement patterns necessary to produce speech sounds when there is no paralysis or weakness of speech muscles. Thought to be due to difficulty with motor planning.**

Figure 4.1 Types of Communicative Disorders Facts and Figures (Reprinted with permission from the Rochester Hearing and Speech Center. http://www.rhsc.org/files/communication-disorders.pdf)

speech sound productions beyond developmental speech errors; this can be characterized by sound substitutions, sound omissions, sound distortions, or other sound errors. *Disorders of fluency* include disturbance in normal flow or rhythm of speech, which can include long pauses between words; frequent repetitions of speech sounds, syllables, words, or phrases; prolongations of speech sounds; and abnormal pauses or stoppages between the syllable of words. Two subtypes of these disorders include: *(a) disorders of nasal resonance:* impaired quality of speech characterized by too little "hyponasality" or too much "hypernasality" nasal airflow. Infants and children with allergies and tonsillar issues are at risk for hyponasality whereas infants with cleft palate are at increased risk of hypernasality related to palatal function and; *(b) disorders of voice or phonation:* impaired quality to speech that can be characterized by aphonia (inability to phonate), impaired phonations (breathy, pitch breaks, hoarse, strained quality), speaking too loud or too softly for speaking conditions, or pitch level that is too high or too low for perceived age and gender. *Disorders of receptive or expressive language* involve language development. Children with special healthcare needs may be at risk in terms of "language development." They may not appropriately understand language, know expected vocabulary, or be able to appropriate combine words to communicate. Silverman (1995) describes people as having a language disorder if they are unable to:

- derive meaning from the words they hear

- derive meaning from the words they read

- formulate and express what they want to say

- formulate and express what they want to write

Pediatric patients are particularly at risk for language delays or impairments related to a variety of factors. Deviations in language production can be observed in children with diagnoses of autism, hearing impairment, and auditory processing disorders, among other conditions.

REFERRAL AND MANAGEMENT: AUDIOLOGISTS AND SPEECH-LANGUAGE PATHOLOGY PROFESSIONS

Most parents are quite perceptive about their children. They may not know the professional jargon to describe differences in their infant or child's ability to hear, speak, understand, interact, or eat, but they know when something is just "not right." If there are concerns noted in early feeding or communication development, a referral to a specialist can help provide answers to the parents' questions.

The professionals who are educated to assess speech and language development and to treat speech and language disorders are called "speech-language pathologists" (sometimes informally referred to as speech therapists or SLPs).

Speech-language pathologists can also help people with swallowing disorders (American Speech-Language Hearing Association, 2012).

Hearing and balance disorders can be assessed, treated, and rehabilitated by an audiologist. Audiologists also select, fit, and dispense amplification systems such as hearing aids; they prevent hearing loss through providing and fitting hearing protective devices, consulting on the effects of noise on hearing, and educating consumers; and they can serve as expert witnesses in litigation related to their areas of expertise. Some audiologists conduct research on hearing, tinnitus, and the balance system (American Speech-Language Hearing Association, 2012).

A referral from a primary healthcare provider is required for an infant or child to be seen by a speech/language pathologist or audiologist. Those seeking services may contact private practitioners, public schools, hospital-based outpatient clinics, college speech clinics, or other specialized community agencies providing these services via licensed professionals. "Speech Referral Guidelines for Pediatrics" are available through the national organization of the American Speech-Language Hearing Association (2012).

An evaluation by a speech/language pathologist will typically involve both informal and formal tests. Formal tests provide developmental norms and standardized test scores to allow for comparison by age and gender. The evaluation may focus on particular area(s) of concern such as receptive language skills, expressive language skills, auditory skills, pragmatics, articulation and phonology, oral motor function for feeding and speech, voice quality, fluency, and critical thinking and reasoning skills "cognitive linguistic function."

Management techniques if deemed warranted may involve individual or group therapy, enrollment in early intervention, and/or therapy in the classroom. Intervention approaches and strategies are dependent on need and should incorporate family-center practices. Intervention strategies may focus on resolution of or compensation for the observed delay or impairment. In the cases of hearing impairment, it must be determined if the issue is temporary or permanent and whether intervention techniques are warranted such as pressure equalization tube placement, cochlear implant, or exploration of the need for hearing aid(s) and/or introduction of manual sign language. There are specific techniques utilized for the various speech and language conditions such as childhood apraxia of speech, dysarthria, orofacial myofunctional disorders, speech sound disorders, stuttering, voice, language-based learning disabilities, preschool language disorders, selective mutism, autism, velopharyngeal incompetence, and brain injury. At times augmentative and/or alternative forms of communication such as voice output devices or picture boards are utilized. For patients with tracheostomies, utilization of a talking valve may be explored.

In conclusion, primary healthcare providers have the opportunity, especially within the context of the medical home, to be the first point of contact when parents have concerns about their child's feeding, communication, overall development, or behavior. The goal of this chapter was to help in recognizing the early symptoms of feeding and communicative challenges so as to best serve in diagnosis, referral, advocacy, and management.

REFERENCES

American Speech-Language Hearing Association. (2012). Information for the Public, Hearing and balance. Retrieved from http://www.asha.org/public/hearing.

Blackman, J.A. (1990). *Medical aspects of developmental disabilities in children birth to three*. Rockville, MD: Aspen.

Hamaguchi, P.M. (2001). Speech, language, and listening: How they develop. In *Childhood speech, language, & listening problems: What every parent should know*. New York, NY: John Wiley & Sons.

Jepsen, C., & Nickel, R.E. (2000). Nutrition and growth. In R.E. Nickel & L.W. Desch (Eds.), *The physician's guide to caring for children with disabilities and chronic conditions*. Baltimore, MD: Paul H. Brookes.

Letcher-Glembo, L. (2000). Craniofacial disorders. In R.E. Nickel & L.W. Desch, *The Physician's Guide to Caring for Children with Disabilities and Chronic Conditions*, Baltimore, MD: Paul H. Brookes.

Roba, C., & Bochacki, V. (1992). Orthodontic considerations. In L. Brodsky, L. Holt, & D.H. Ritter-Schmidt (Eds.), *Craniofacial anomalies: An interdisciplinary approach*, St. Louis, MO: Mosby-Year Book.

Shipley, K.G., & McAfee, J.G. (2009). *Assessment in speech-language pathology*. Clifton Park, NY: Delmar Cengage Learning.

Silverman, S.H. (1995). *Human communication disorders: An introduction* (4th ed.). New York, NY: Merrill/ Macmillan.

Volk, M.S., Arnold, S., & Brodsky, L. (1992). Otolaryngology and audiology. In L. Brodsky, L. Holt, & D.H. Ritter-Schmidt (Eds.), *Craniofacial anomalies: An interdisciplinary approach*, St. Louis: Mosby-Year Book.

CHAPTER 5

CARING FOR CHILDREN WITH MOBILITY DIFFERENCES

Jeannine Roth

Caring for Children with Special Healthcare Needs and Their Families: A Handbook for Healthcare Professionals, First Edition. Edited by Linda L. Eddy.
© 2013 John Wiley & Sons, Inc. Published 2013 by John Wiley & Sons, Inc.

WHAT IS MOBILITY?

For the purposes of this chapter, mobility will be defined as "the state or quality of movement (Thomas, 1997, p. 1139). For children with special needs such as cerebral palsy, spina bifida, and other musculoskeletal disabilities, mobility can impede participation in everyday life. Think about the care for a child with one of the above diagnoses and the mobility orders that are written while in the hospital: ambulate three times a day, up out of bed three times a day for 30 minutes, or up to wheelchair three times a day. These medical orders are common and help to improve respiratory function and help to progress the patient to discharge. However, there is more to mobility for children with special needs than maintaining and returning to baseline mobility after a hospitalization. Throughout this chapter the above definition of mobility will be combined with the international classification of functioning, disability, and health (ICF) to demonstrate the importance of mobility, how assistive devices impact mobility, and how healthcare professionals can help promote preventative health through mobility.

The International Classification of Functioning, Disability and Health (ICF)

The ICF definition of "mobility" includes health, body, and societal perspectives. When addressing the body, we are concerned about structure and function, or: at what level is the individual able to move, and what limitations are found? "Function" includes not only quality of movement, but how well the body can function in a particular child's environment and the child's ability to interact and move within that environment. Another important aspect of the ICF definition is the individual's ability to participate in the activities that are important to him or her (http://www.who.int/classifications/icf/en/). For children mobility and play is a major part of their lives; it is how they learn and master skills (Wilson, Ahmann, & Wong, 1998). As healthcare providers we need to promote mobility not only in the sense of the body being able to function to meet activities of daily living (ADLs), but to enable children with special needs to optimize their functional ability within their environment and within their social network. When functional ability is optimized a child's potential for optimal health is not only realized physically, but mentally and socially as well.

According to the World Health Organization (WHO), health "is a state of complete physical, mental and social well being and not merely the absence of disease or infirmity" (Thorpe, 2009). The definition provided by WHO can be used to help healthcare professionals understand that there is more to mobility for children with special needs than a child's physical ability or lack of mobility. The definition of "health" will be different for each individual, especially for those with a chronic health condition. When adults with cerebral palsy (CP) were interviewed about their general state of health, they considered themselves healthy, even though they were not free from disease or infirmary (Thorpe, 2009). Although measuring quality of life for children with disabilities is difficult, it may be a bit easier in the area of mobility. Quality of life related to mobility relates to one's ability to be active or participate in desired activities (Thorpe). Therefore, participation is a key component to health (Imms, 2008). The WHO defines participation as "involvement in a life situation (Imms, p. 1867). For children with special needs, involvement or participation in life situations is very dependent on their functional ability, which takes into account their body structure and the ability of the body to accommodate movement. For a child who is wheelchair-bound, participation in some activities such as going on rides at an amusement park may not be possible, but creativity on the part of healthcare team members can help these children find satisfying alternative experiences. Remember that there is more to health than just being free from disease or a chronic condition. For children with special needs, being free from chronic conditions may not be possible, but the healthcare team can plan and advocate with the family to offer as many inclusive activities as possible.

The ways in which having a special healthcare need affects participation, including social participation, needs to be taken into consideration. For children with special needs, function and quality of life (QOL) are commonly clumped together. Even though one can have a direct effect on the other, QOL is a multidimensional concept that not only includes function, but also psychological state, cognitive ability, social interaction, social, physical and emotional functioning (Shelly et al., 2008). Therefore, a child with special needs may have high-level physical functioning, but may be unable to participate in particular activities due to impaired cognitive or emotional functioning. Thus, inability to participate in activities may be separate from impaired mobility.

PARTICIPATION AND FUNCTIONAL ABILITY

The child's functional level is determined, in part, by his or her diagnosis. Children with mobility issues may use one or more forms of assistive devices to optimize their mobility. For children with cerebral palsy (CP), bodily function related to mobility is measured using the Gross Motor Functional Classification System (GMFCS).

This system helps healthcare providers determine how independent children are in their ability to move about in their environment. As shown in Table 5.1, the higher the level of gross motor functioning classification, the more assistance is needed and the more dependent the child is on help with mobility.

CARING FOR CHILDREN WITH
MOBILITY DIFFERENCES

Table 5.1

LEVEL I – Walks without Limitations
LEVEL II – Walks with Limitations
LEVEL III – Walks Using a Hand-Held Mobility Device
LEVEL IV – Self-Mobility with Limitations; May Use Powered Mobility
LEVEL V – Transported in a Manual Wheelchair

Distinctions Between Levels I and II – Compared with children and youth in Level I, children and youth in Level II have limitations walking long distances and balancing; may need a hand-held mobility device when first learning to walk; may use wheeled mobility when traveling long distances outdoors and in the community; require the use of a railing to walk up and down stairs; and are not as capable of running and jumping.
Distinctions Between Levels II and III – Children and youth in Level II are capable of walking without a hand-held mobility device after age 4 (although they may choose to use one at times). Children and youth in Level III need a hand-held mobility device to walk indoors and use wheeled mobility outdoors and in the community.
Distinctions Between Levels III and IV – Children and youth in Level III sit on their own or require at most limited external support to sit, are more independent in standing transfers, and walk with a hand-held mobility device. Children and youth in Level IV function in sitting (usually supported) but self-mobility is limited. Children and youth in Level IV are more likely to be transported in a manual wheelchair or use powered mobility.
Distinctions Between Levels IV and V – Children and youth in Level V have severe limitations in head and trunk control and require extensive assisted technology and physical assistance. Self-mobility is achieved only if the child/youth can learn how to operate a powered wheelchair.

From the article of: GMFCS © Robert Palisano, Peter Rosenbaum, Stephen Walter, Dianne Russell, Ellen Wood, Barbara Galuppi, 1997
CanChild Centre for Childhood Disability Research, McMaster University
(Reference: Dev Med Child Neurol 1997;39:214–223)

Being confined to a wheelchair affects a child's ability to move around his or her environment and participate in life situations. A child with CP and a GMCFS classification of level III or IV has self-mobility with limitations; he or she may use a powered wheelchair (Rosenbaum et al. 2008). The use of a powered wheelchair enables the child to move around his or her environment, but may not allow full participation in activities that the child or adolescent desires. This is due, in part, to barriers created by society.

Children with disabilities do not participate in recreational or physical activities as much as do their nondisabled peers (Majnemer et al., 2008). When examining the reasons for this decreased participation, contributing factors include more energy expenditure than nondisabled peers (Voorman et al., 2006), limited functional ability (Fowler et al., 2007) and lack of availability of programs for children with special needs in the community (Fowler et al.). This research demonstrates that it is important for healthcare providers to figure out how to promote some type of physical activity for children with disabilities in order to promote mobility and improve overall physical fitness and health. For example, there are many programs throughout the United States that enable children with disabilities to participate in physical activities. One such program is the Hospital Special Program (HSP), which is run through The Children's Hospital in Denver, Colorado. The HSP at Denver's Children Hospital enables children with a variety of disabilities to participate in both winter and summer sports. The focus of the winter sports is skiing; the focus of the summer sports is golf and tennis. These activities allow children to learn a sport, become active, and increase physical fitness, and also provide them with a social network in which to share experiences with peers. Children with disabilities are more likely to participate in physical activities by themselves or with family members (Chow & Fung, 2005) than with peers, and participation decreases as children enter adolescence (Bruton & Bartlett, 2010). Children learn through play, and it is important for healthcare providers to remember that play is a key component to normal growth and development (Dickinson, Parkinson, Ravens-Sieberer, & Schirripa, 2007) that will also help to promote mobility for all children of all functional levels.

Being able to get around their environment is one of the greatest challenges noted by both adults and children with disabilities (Young et al., 2007). Take a moment and think about your activities for the day: did you have to walk down stairs to get to your car? Was there snow covering the sidewalk or a curb that you had to step down? Lastly, did you stop for coffee, and the counter was high or the coffee shop was small and narrow? These environmental barriers go unnoticed by those of us who do not have a disability or use assistive devices to get around. However, for children with impaired mobility these barriers limit the amount and types of activities that are available to them.

Activities requiring mobility are particularly hard for children with GMCFS of III, IV and V (Palisano et al., 2009) or those who use any assistive device. When examining how the use of assistive devices impacts a child's ability to be mobile, it is important to understand the social model of disability. The social model reminds us that disabled people have the same desires, needs, and aspirations of nondisabled people(Bennett, 2011).

In 2009 a study on rehabilitation services suggested that services based on the social model could help optimize children's participation in home, school, and community life (Palisano et al., 2009), a very different view than the medical model healthcare providers often work from that focuses on the impairment limiting the child's ability to be mobile. This difference in thinking can sometimes limit how healthcare providers think about mobility for children with disabilities. For example, for children with spina bifida, their impairment affects not only their mobility, but usually also their genitourinary system and gastrointestinal system. Therefore, as healthcare providers we are focusing on the impairments and how to make the children as healthy as possible, not necessarily on their ability to be mobile and participate fully within their community. However, the advantages of looking beyond the medical model and embracing full participation has health benefits too. For example, children and adolescents with spina bifida are at risk for obesity due to lack of physical activity and poor level of fitness (Borg-Emons et al., 2003). An important question to ask as healthcare providers is this: is this risk for obesity and subnormal level of fitness (Borg-Emons et al.) due to the impairment or the lack of mobility for these children? Is our focus on the impairment blurring our judgment about how mobile these children can be? As healthcare providers, we have the opportunity to increase mobility and health.

As mentioned earlier in the chapter, the HSP program is a great example of helping children with spina bifida gain perspective about their abilities. In this program, mobility is promoted through sports and play. These children have ski instructors and coaches who enable them to participate to their full ability. Programs such as these focus on ability instead of inability (Crow, 1996).

Assistive technology

Full participation in activities is aided, in part, by use of assistive technology. Assistive technology can be as simple as a cane to help with balance or as complex as a technological gait analysis that enables orthopedic surgeons to identify precisely what muscles or bones need correction to optimize mobility. Assessment for assistive devices requires understanding what the least-intrusive aid is that will enable the child or adolescent to participate in activities.

For one teen with cerebral palsy, assistive technology enables her to go to high school and attend classes with her nondisabled friends. Stephanie, a high school junior who attends a large city school, uses a wide variety of assistive technology to enable her to be mobile. Her cerebral palsy affects both of her legs, and her GMFCS classification is level III. Stephanie utilizes a scooter while at school, along with crutches. At home she has a walker and crutches to get around. While out in the community it is Stephanie's goal to walk with only crutches. Her ultimate goal is to walk across the stage at graduation without any assistive devices. Stephanie's story is not unusual. For healthcare providers and especially nurses, it seems that families are always asking what we think about this new device or this new test. Sometimes the answers are easy, and at other times there seems to be no simple one. However, it is clear that advances in technology offer enhanced mobility for many children with disabilities.

Gait analysis

Making ambulation and mobility a possibility or optimizing mobility for individuals such as Stephanie is the goal of gait analysis. Before the advent of gait analysis technology, most decisions on what medical interventions needed to be done were based on the clinical history and physical examination. Today, orthopedic surgeons not only review the clinical history, they assess family dynamics and support resources that are available to the families in order to help promote success of musculoskeletal surgery (Davids, Ounpuu, DeLuca, & Davis, 2003). For children who undergo a gait analysis, the procedure enables surgeons to see skeletal abnormalities more precisely, such as hip angle and hip movement. The analysis is video recorded on high speed motion-picture cameras with reflective markers on the surface of the skin; these markers along with the recording provide a way to define motion, see how the body is compensating for weak muscles, and decide which muscles are not working up to their potential and which ones are working too much (Davids et al.). Once the analysis is complete, a team of providers including the surgeon, physical therapist, and bioengineer will meet to discuss what would be the best treatment options for the child. One of the most important aspects is what the goal is for that patient. Gait analysis can identify multiple areas that may need surgical intervention, but not all of them need to be done to meet the goals of that particular person. It is also essential to note that every surgical intervention has risks and benefits. Even though the goal of utilizing this assistive technology is to improve the patient lives, sometimes assistive technology can be overwhelming for both the providers, families, and patients. Therefore, it is important to realize that not every child with a musculoskeletal disability needs every possible assistive technology.

WHAT CAN NURSES DO TO HELP CHILDREN WITH DISABILITIES?

Nurses are in a unique position to embrace both the medical model to help meet the complex health needs of children with disabilities and the social model to help children and families achieve optimal participation in the community. The Health Belief Model (Pender, 2006) helps nurses and other healthcare providers individualize care for children and families.

Central to the model is the importance of individual characteristics and experiences. One child with a disability may have the same diagnosis as another child but have very different personal characteristics, past experiences, and goals for the future. Remember Stephanie, the junior high school student whose goal was to walk without any assistive devices at graduation? Her personal characteristics include a strong inner drive and a very supportive family who push her to reach her goals and to be independent. Previous experiences related to her ultimate goal of walking independently included orthopedic surgeons telling her and her family that she would never walk. Her family did not believe this and told the doctor they would see him for postoperative follow-up and Stephanie would be walking into his office in some fashion. Since that experience she has worked diligently with her physical therapist and two separate orthopedic surgeons to reach her goal. When Stephanie was asked if she thought she could meet that goal, she stated: "my physical therapist will never let me not meet my goal. Dan and I have a connection that helps him push me to that next level." The treatment program for Stephanie is possible because she has both support and an inner drive to reach her goal. Stephanie's goal is possible because she can see herself walking across the stage at graduation, and each day she completes her physical therapy she feels stronger. The barriers for Stephanie are few: she states that her "whole school supports her goal", especially after her story was featured in the school newspaper. In applying the HPM to Stephanie, she has high self–efficacy about her ability to reach her goal(Pender, 2006). She is able to commit to her goal, and to juggle the demands of high school and her increased physical therapy schedule.

CONCLUSION

Mobility is so much more than being able to walk: it is finding a way to participate as fully as possible in desired activities and feeling like goals are attainable. We as healthcare providers can make a difference in the lives of children and adolescents with mobility impairments by focusing not on what the child cannot do, but what he or she can do if societal attitudes and barriers are removed.

REFERENCES

Bennett, S. (2011). Living with cerebral palsy. Retrieved from http://www.livingwithcerebralpalsy.com/index.php

Borg-Emons, H.J.G.v.d., Bussmann, J.B.J., Meyerink, H.J., et al. (2003). Body fat, fitness and level of everyday physical activity in adolescents and young adults with meningomyelocele. *Journal of Rehabilitative Medicine*, *35*, 271–275.

Bruton, L., & Bartlett, D. (2010). Description of exercise particpation of adolescents with cerebral palsy across a 4-year period. *Pediatric Physical Therapy*, 180–188.

Chow, B., & Fung, L. (2005). Correlates of children's physical activity, and physical self-perceptions. *Research Quarterly for Exercise and Sport*, *76*(1), 103–104.

Crow, L. (1996). Including all of our lives: Renewing the social model of disability. *Disability and Illness: Exploring the Divide, Disability Press and Reader Inclusive Education: Diverse Perspective*, 1–15.

Davids, J., Ounpuu, S., DeLuca, P., & Davis, R. (2003). Optimization of walking ability of children with cerebral palsy. *The Journal of Bone & Joint Surgery, 85-A*(11), 2224–2234.

Dickinson, H.O., Parkinson, K.N., Ravens-Sieberer, U., & Schirripa, G. (2007). Self-reported quality of life of 8–12-year-old children with cerebral palsy: A cross-sectional European study. *The Lancet, 369*(9580), 2171–2180.

Fowler, E.G., Kolobe, T.H., Damiano, D.L., et al. (2007). Promotion of physical fitness and prevention of secondary conditions for children with cerebral palsy: Section on Pediatrics Research Summit Proceedings. *Physical Therapy, 87*(11), 1495–1510.

Imms, C. (2008). Children with cerebral palsy participate: A review of the literature. *Disability and Rehabilitation, 10*(24), 1867–1884.

Majnemer, A., Shevell, M., Law, M., et al. (2008). Participation and enjoyment of leisure activities in school-aged children with cerebral palsy. *Developmental Medicine and Child Neurology, 50*, 751–758.

Palisano, R., Kang, L.-J., Chiarello, L., et al. (2009). Social and community participation of children and youth with cerebral palsy is associated with age and gross motor function classification. *Physical Therapy, 89*(12), 1304–1314.

Pender, N. (2006). University of Michigan School of Nursing. Retrieved from http://currentnursing.com/nursing_theory/health_promotion_model.htm

Rosenbaum, P.L., Palisano, R.J., Bartlett, D.J., et al.(2008). Development of the Gross Motor Function Classification System for cerebral palsy. *Developmental Medicine and Child Neurology, 50*(4), 249–253.

Shelly, A., Davis, E., Waters, E., et al. (2008). The relationship between quality of life and functioning for children with cerebral palsy. *Developmental Medicine and Child Neurology, 50*(3), 199–203.

Thomas, C.L. (Ed.). (1997) *Taber's cyclopedic medical dictionary* (18th ed.). Philadelphia, PA: F.A. Davis.

Thorpe, D. (2009). The role of fitness in health and disease: status of adults with cerebral palsy. *Developmental Medicine and Child Neurology, 51*(s4), 52–58.

Voorman, J., Dallmeijer, A., Schuengel, C., et al. (2006). Activities and participation of 9–13 year-old child with cerebral palsy. *Clinical Rehabilitation 20*, 937–948.

Wilson, D., Ahmann, E. & Wong, D.L. (1998). *Whaley & Wong's nursing care of infants and children*. (p. 161).(6th ed.). St. Louis: Mosby.

Young, B., Rice, H., Dixon-Woods, M., et al. (2007). A qualitative study of the health-related quality of life of disabled children. *Developmental Medicine and Child Neurology, 49*(9), 660–665.

CHAPTER 6

CARING FOR THE CHILD WITH SPECIAL SOCIAL AND EMOTIONAL NEEDS

Sheela M. Choppala-Nestor with Portia Riley

INTRODUCTION

The ability to have and maintain social and emotional connections is central to the human experience. Interpersonal interaction is, in fact, critical for human development. Erickson, Sullivan, and Winnicott, among others, eloquently explain the critical role of healthy childhood relationships to the experience of a healthy adulthood (Mitchell & Black, 1995). Therefore, difficulties with social or emotional functioning must be identified early and addressed effectively for the sake of life success. According to Kessler et al. (2005) half of all lifetime mental disorders in the United States occur before the age of 14, thus underscoring the need for nurses to be alert to mental illness in youth.

It is important to distinguish between a temporary alteration in functioning and psychopathology. A child may experience a phase of troubled or difficult behavior in response to a situational stressor. Psychopathology, however, is more enduring and results in the breakdown of social functioning and school functioning with far-reaching effects.

This chapter focuses on child psychopathology. Psychiatric disorders in children and teens are often difficult to identify, understand, and treat. Pediatric nurses may be among the first individuals outside the child's family to notice emotional and behavioral trouble. This chapter is intended to help nurses understand the picture being painted by their assessment and to help develop a plan of intervention for the child and the child's family.

CARING FOR THE CHILD WITH
SPECIAL SOCIAL AND EMOTIONAL
NEEDS

STRUCTURE OF THIS CHAPTER

The information in this chapter is presented as a general guide to working with children with psychiatric problems. Etiologies of child and adolescent mental illness are briefly discussed before the presentation of a practical approach to child assessment. Interventions and resources for nurses or families are then discussed. This chapter also includes selected case studies of frequently seen psychiatric conditions to illustrate the assessment and intervention processes described.

ETIOLOGICAL THEORIES

In children and adolescents there are many factors that contribute to the development of mental disease. The complex interface of these factors often makes it difficult to pinpoint a single etiological cause (Mash & Dozois, 2003; Colson, 2006). For example, not every child with a parent with mental illness will develop mental illness, and not every child who experiences a difficult social environment will be disordered. Yet, there are known contributors to mental illness. Some include:

- Genetics and Neurobiology – Twin studies demonstrate the heritability of psychiatric illness, including anxiety disorders, mood disorders, schizophrenia, ADHD, and even autism (Kaplan & Saddock, 2009; Bailey et al., 1995). Technological advances have enabled researchers to find the genetic mechanisms that impact child psychopathology (Lombroso, Pauls & Leckman, 1994). Neuroimaging has also implicated regions of the brain involved in mental illness. Hyperactivity or hypoactivity in areas of the brain can often explain dysfunctional behaviors. Anatomical abnormalities are also associated with illnesses such as schizophrenia (Kaplan & Saddock).

- Temperament – Thomas, Chess, and Birch (1965) produced seminal research that identified three child temperament types. They were able to show that there are nine characteristics that are demonstrated universally by children. In rating children's responsiveness to situations illuminating the nine characteristics, they developed the classification of the following temperaments: easy, slow-to-warm-up, and difficult. It has been shown that higher rates of diagnosable behavioral trouble occur in those with a difficult temperament whereas lower rates occur in those with an easy temperament despite environmental influences.

- Attachment and Maltreatment – A child develops a sense of self and also a sense of others during the early stages of life. Many theorists posit that healthy attachment and security is the basis for stress reduction (Mash & Dozois, 2003). Conversely, maltreated children experience distinct changes in the stress-regulating fields of their brains that cause vulnerability and demonstrate a connection to disordered behavior (Hart, Gunnar, & Cicacchetti, 1995; Eckendrode et al., 2001).

- Environmental stress – This mostly involves issues with the social environment. Some risk factors for children include low socioeconomic status, parent criminality, and severe discord between parents. Overcrowding and problems with physical safety are also environmental stresses that impact development and can lead to mental dysfunction (Colson, 2006). Poverty is a leading risk factor for abuse and neglect.

- Cognitive Dysfunction – According to Mash and Dozois (2003) who summarized the cognitive literature, cognitive frameworks are set early in life from the child's experiences. The child then perceives and interprets events and feelings through that framework. Depressive or anxious frameworks can lead to negative patterns of thinking and then result in negative behaviors. Additionally, cognitive *deficits* can lead to impulsive behaviors.

- Cultural isolation or dissonance – Minority children face additional risks. In addition to marginalization, it has been shown that minority children lack cultural role models, and experience the stress of having different cultural expectations. This puts them at risk for developing mental and emotional problems (Yeh et al., 2004).

THE PROCESS OF CHILD ASSESSMENT AND INTERVENTION

Much like all that we do in nursing, effectively helping children with special social and emotional needs involves a process. The process of caring for a child with social and emotional needs includes assessing the child and family, assessing systems associated with the child, and analyzing the data gathered, and then proceeding to intervene in an evidenced-based and emotionally sensitive way.

The salience of rapport building to the process

The importance of engagement with the child and family with social and emotional needs cannot be underestimated. Trustworthiness, authenticity, and clear communication are the basis for strong engagement.

Communication is the single most important factor under your control when it comes to gathering data through an interview. The assessment of a child's emotional state rests on successful interaction with both the child and secondary sources. Communicating requires empathy, sensitivity, and skill. The child interview must be tailored to the needs of the child. Understanding human development will help you strategize the session based on the emotional and cognitive abilities of the child (Sadock & Sadock, 2007). Based on the child's age and needs, parents may or may not be present for the initial interview. The impact of parents' presence or absence is important to conclusions made about the interview and the content that emerges.

McConaughy (2005) provides information on the details of conducting the interview. Some of her suggestions include:

- Assure the child that he or she is not stupid, crazy, or being punished

- Maintain a semi-structured interview in language understandable to the child; allow flexibility in sequencing of topics but assure that all information is gathered

- Ensure that the setting is comfortable, not intimidating, and that the child and interviewer are more or less on the same physical plane (to reduce any implication of authority by the interviewer)

- Provide the child information about the purpose and format of the interview

- Prior to the start of the body of the interview, provide information on confidentiality and the limits of confidentiality (i.e., tell the child that you will discuss with him or her the information that others may see in written reports, and ask the child how he or she may want that information presented to others). Also let the child know that dangerous situations are exceptional situations in which you may have to talk to others because you want to keep the child safe.

- Questioning strategies are based on the cognitive abilities of the child. Open-ended questions should be connected to contexts that are familiar to the child (i.e., ask the child about games he or she plays at recess or how the child does on homework).

Taffel (2010) stresses the importance of approaching teens in a respectful manner by avoiding treating them like children. He says that if we routinely interact with teens, it may be helpful to understand their lives by asking them questions about their interests and teen culture. He also talks about the fact that teens must be approached under the assumption that they *do* know what is missing from their lives and are open to helper questions that are genuine and based in a desire to help. Based on Taffel's information questions that open the door to teens revealing their concerns include:

- "How can I help you?"

- "What would you like to change about yourself or your life?"

- "If you could have three wishes, what would they be?" (This question is also highly effective in preteens.)

It also important to be clear about the reality and limitations of what you are able to do for them. This transparency is the foundation of the therapeutic relationship.

Systematic data gathering

The primary source for data is generally the child or adolescent who is having difficulty. However, in the assessment of children secondary sources are often critical (Varcarolis, 2006). Secondary sources are parents or caregivers, other

CARING FOR THE CHILD WITH
SPECIAL SOCIAL AND EMOTIONAL
NEEDS

family members, and teachers. Although a semi-structured interview is often the starting point of the assessment, other data collection methods include observation, a physical exam and, structured questionnaires.

The semi-structured interview covers the following regions:

- History of present illness, including chief complaint, current symptoms, and results of previous care

- Developmental history, including maternal pregnancy history

- Educational history and school issues

- Social history, including peer relationships and adult relationships

- Cultural identification, including race, ethnicity, and religion

- Medical history, including issues with the healthcare system

- Substance use history

- Family history of psychiatric and mental health problems

- Family structure, dynamics, and communication patterns (this is likely a good place to ask whether the child has experienced any physical, sexual, or emotional abuse or neglect)

- Socioeconomic status and possible financial stressors

- Cultural identification and impact of culture on family dynamic

- Strengths, including hobbies, skills, and extracurricular activities

- Support systems, including extended family, friends, spiritual/ religious connections, and group affiliations (Colson, 2006; Morrison, 2001)

During the interview you will be gathering observational data. Observations are best organized in the format of the mental status examination. Just like the adult psychiatric examination, elements of mental status include appearance, behavior during the interview, psychomotor status, speech rate, thought processes, thought content, judgment, and insight. Note any incongruencies between reported data and observed data.

By the time you are done with the interview, you will be able to determine whether it is beneficial to proceed with additional data collection through

Table 6.1 Child Behavior Tools

Tool		Access Information
Child Behavior Checklist (CBCL)	Also called the Achenbach, this is a checklist, which means that it is not diagnostic but gives you data on a child's behavior that can help identify maladaptive functioning (Achenbach & Ruffle, 2000). It is extensively studied and can be correlated to DSM-IV diagnoses (Achenbach, 2011). / This can help with measuring post-treatment effects and changes over time. Specialized versions can be rated by parent, teachers, clinicians, and youth.	http://www.aseba.org/ Must be purchased
Conners 3	Although it captures data on a wide number of symptoms, it has been known for its ability to detect Attention Deficit and Hyperactivity Disorder (Conners, 2004–2012).	http://www.mhs.com/ Must be purchased
Center for Epidemiological Studies Depression Scale Modified for Children (CES-DC)	This is best used for detecting mood problems in children age 6–17 (Center for Epidemiological Studies Depression Scale for Children, n.d). It is short, easy to administer and score.	http://www.brightfutu res.org/mentalhealth/ pdf/tools.html Available free

An invaluable summary of child and adolescent checklists, questionnaires, and surveys that cover multiple diagnoses can be found at http://www2.massgeneral.org/schoolpsychiatry/checklists_table .asp and http://www2.massgeneral.org/schoolpsychiatry/schoolpsychiatry_screeningtools.asp
Source: American Psychiatric Association. (2000). Diagnostic and statistical manual of mental disorders DSM-IV TR fourth edition. American Psychiatric Publishing: Arlington, VA.

structured questionnaires. Although questionnaires may help quantify your findings, most instruments that have been extensively studied and have proven reliability and validity must be purchased. Costs can often restrict their ability to be widely used if you have a limited budget. Table 6.1 lists three frequently used questionnaires and where you can find them.

Analysis of data gathered

Once data has been gathered some conclusions should be drawn about the child's mental health. It is important to accurately diagnose in order to accurately intervene and support the child. Although providing a psychiatric diagnosis is the responsibility of a medical provider, nurses can decide on the next

Table 6.2 Stages of Development

Developmental Stage	Psychosocial Crisis	Developmental Task
Infancy	Trust vs. mistrust	Attachment to parent – If successful the individual will be able to form trusting and healthy relationships throughout his or her lifetime.
Early childhood	Autonomy vs. shame and doubt	Basic self-control and confidence in environmental exploration – If successful the individual will be able to cultivate self-confidence and independence.
Late childhood	Initiative vs. guilt	Sense of purpose – Successful resolution results in self-directedness in activities.
School age	Industry vs. inferiority	Competence in tasks – If successful the individual will be able to feel pride in accomplishing his or her work and not fear comparison to others.
Adolescence	Identity vs. role confusion	Formation of identity – Individuals who are successful at this developmental stage achieve a sense of identity and confidence about who they are that later enables them to develop intimacy.

Adapted from Carson, V., & Trubowitz, J. (2006). Relevant theories and therapies for nursing practice. *In E. Varcarolis, V. Benner, & N. Shoemaker (Eds.),* Foundations of psychiatric and mental health nursing: A clinical approach (pp. 15–33). St. Louis, MO: Saunders Elsevier.

CARING FOR THE CHILD WITH SPECIAL SOCIAL AND EMOTIONAL NEEDS

step of care based on whether they believe a psychiatric diagnosis is apparent. Here are some steps that can help with this process:

- Determine the child's developmental level and conclude whether the child's social and emotional development is appropriate to his or her age. Table 6.2 depicts Erickson's stages of psychosocial development. This model provides an age-based guide to the social and psychological development of individuals, positing that at each stage of development all of us experience a crisis on which our development hinges. Although this model has suffered some critique for its Western-centric base, it still remains effective as a general guide for assessing child development. Remember that cultural experts must be used as part of your team to ensure that behaviors are evaluated against the cultural norms of the individual.

- If there is a high degree of suspicion that the child has a clinical psychiatric disorder, obtain a formal psychiatric evaluation and diagnosis. Within Box 6.1 are listed disorders first evident in children and adolescents according to the *Diagnostic and Statistical Manual of Mental Disorders IV-Text Revision (DSM IV-TR)* (American Psychiatric Association, 2000).

- If a psychiatric disorder does not exist, determine the stressor causing the problem behavior; issues that could play a salient role include family problems, healthcare system problems, economic problems, social problems, and/or educational problems

---

Box 6.1 Disorders Usually First Diagnosed in Infancy, Childhood or Adolescence. *Full excerpt can be found in the* American Psychiatric Association, *Diagnostic and Statistical Manual of Mental Disorders* (4th ed., text rev. 2000)(*DSM-IV-TR*) Washington, DC: American Psychiatric Association.

Mental Retardation (mild, moderate, severe or profound)
Learning Disorders (reading, mathematics, written expression)
Developmental Coordination Disorder
Communication Disorders (expressive language, mixed receptive-expressive language, phonological or stuttering)
Pervasive Developmental Disorders (autistic, Rett's, childhood disintegrative, Asperger's)
Attention Deficit and Hyperactivity Disorders (inattentive, hyperactive-impulsive, conduct disorder, oppositional defiant, disruptive behavior not otherwise specified)
Feeding and Eating Disorders of Infancy or Early Childhood (pica, rumination disorder, feeding disorder)
Tic Disorders (Tourette's, chronic motor or vocal tic, transient tic)
Elimination Disorders (encopresis, enuresis)
Separation Anxiety Disorder
Selective Mutism
Reactive Attachment Disorder
Stereotypic Movement Disorder

Note: Each category generally has a diagnosis that captures a disorder that does not meet the criteria for the more specific diagnoses; it is called a "not otherwise specified" diagnosis

---

Intervention

Interventional strategies will vary based on resources available in your community. Here are some steps to take when embarking on this phase of the process:

- Share your conclusions with the child and family

- Obtain their perspective and find out whether they agree with your conclusions; if they disagree, find out if they have more data to share with you

- Develop a multidisciplinary treatment team based on the diagnoses and/or issues identified

- Develop goals with the child and the child's family. An interdisciplinary intervention plan can only be successful if the child, family, and team agree on outcomes and together work toward achieving those outcomes.

THE INTERDISCIPLINARY TEAM: A CRITICAL ASPECT OF THE INTERVENTION

Depending on your community and the community resources available to you, developing a multidisciplinary team may be challenging. A psychiatric specialist (medical doctor (MD), nurse practitioner (NP), or physician's assistant (PA)) is ultimately responsible for determining diagnosis. In communities that do not have a specialist, the diagnosis may be made by a primary care provider.

The ideal team consists of a board certified psychiatric provider (MD, NP, or PA), a marriage-family therapist or licensed social worker, and a case manager. Culturally responsive teams have language interpreters. A functional team also includes you, the nurse who operates as the community and/or family liaison, and/or the person assisting the family in successfully building skills.

Many agencies have teams already formed so you may only need to find the agency in your area that has a functioning one. In communities where child-oriented agencies do not exist, you may have to piece together the team and act as its coordinator.

CASE REVIEWS OF SELECT DISORDERS

In this section some select disorders are discussed and exemplars provided. A few of these disorders have been selected because of their prevalence (autism, social phobia, and major depressive disorder). An exemplar and discussion of anorexia is also included because it can be easily overlooked as "just a phase."

Autism Spectrum Disorders (ASDs)

According to the Centers for Disease Control (CDC) the identification of children who meet criteria for a disorder in the autism spectrum is on the rise. The most recent data indicates that autism statistics varies across the country; the prevalence of ASDs in 8 year old children ranges from 1 in 47 to 1 in 210

(CDC, 2012). To date there is no cure for ASDs but there are interventions to help children and families.

Joey is a 7-year-old Vietnamese male brought in by his parents because he has a coin fascination, which makes it difficult to take him anywhere that there will be an exchange of money. Joey is nonverbal, and is unable to behave appropriately in most settings. Joey has been known to dive behind counters in stores trying to obtain coins from people or tills. His increasing strength has made it difficult to manage his behavior in public. His parents have to take him places because of childcare issues so they attempted to teach him social skills but Joey seems to be unable to learn them. School issues prompted the family to seek help. When his family is unable to figure out what he is trying to communicate, he engages in hitting his head, scratching himself on the face, and throwing himself on the floor or against the wall. His parents are embarrassed and feel deep shame because of his behavior. They are also frustrated due to being unable to understand Joey's special needs. They themselves face a cultural and language barrier. Joey has a 10-year-old sister who he responds to. She is able to calm him down so she is often in the position of managing Joey and helping her parents with language issues. Even his sister is unable to redirect him when coins are involved. The family does not know where to go for help.

Impressions. Joey's stereotyped behavior, lack of communication skills, and general lack of social connectedness indicate that he has an ASD. His condition is further complicated by the presence of a coin obsession. Comorbid conditions are not uncommon with ASDs. Joey's family are challenged not just by his behavior, but by cultural and language issues as well. The family dynamic places a burden on Joey's sister, which could impact her development as well.

Interventions. In Joey's case a multidisciplinary team was most useful. A medical provider diagnosed him and prescribed medication for his obsessiveness. The nurse coordinating the team sought a cultural specialist who helped bridge the language barrier and helped her provide psychoeducation concerning Joey's diagnosis. The therapist on the team utilized the help of the cultural specialist to sensitively address the shame issues, the family dynamic, and the maintaining of the child development needs of both Joey and his sister. The team's coordinating nurse was also able to engage team members to help with some of Joey's specific issues. A specialized speech therapist assisted Joey learn basic forms of communication.

Although unavailable in Joey's community, special educational programs do exist specifically for the ASD population. These are ideal and provide not only an appropriate environment for autistic children to learn and develop skills, but a respite for the family as well. Some communities have pure respite programs designed for families of this population.

Resources. A credible and condensed source of information is provided by the National Institute of Mental Health at www.ncbi.nlm.nih.gov/pubmedhe alth/PMH0002494/. The CDC provides information about autism in general and additionally provides state by state prevalence data at www.cdc.gov/ ncbddd/autism/index.html. You can find national and local resources for children and families by going to www.autismspeaks.org.

Social phobia

Social phobia is significant because of the disruption it can cause in a child's school life. According to Merikagas et al. (2010) 5.5% of 13–18 year olds in this country suffer from social phobia. The child and adolescent mental health web site of Massachusetts General Hospital reflects a concern: social phobia may be under-recognized in younger children as their behavior may be dismissed as being part of a shy personality when in reality their self-consciousness around being watched or judged causes pathological distress. Although social phobia is more prevalent in females, it affects males as well, and is both persistent and impairing both persistent and impairing (Burstein et al., 2011).

David is a 15-year-old white male high school student. When he was young his mother noticed that he seemed to be very shy around others. He often seemed quieter in public than at home. At the beginning of middle school he told his mother that he didn't want to go to a new school and was sure that people there would think he was "dumb" because he never knew what to say when the teacher called on him. His mother stressed that he just needed to be strong and act like the rest of the kids in his class. David tried but he could barely make eye contact with the other kids. He only spoke to those kids whom he knew from elementary school. He began having stomach aches and often missed school or came home early. Although he did well when he actually did homework, he was absent too often to stay abreast of his coursework and he was barely passing his classes. When his father left his mother for another woman, David's phobia worsened. He attended school even less. His mother did not have the emotional energy or time to ask David about his experience. His frequent absences from school and his failing grades led school officials to contact his mother. She was upset with David and wanted him to overcome his shyness. She even wondered if he missed school because of laziness. At the prompting of his school counselor she took him to a mental health center for evaluation.

Impressions. David displayed intense anxiety that primarily manifested in discomfort around others and a feeling that he was being evaluated. Although he attempted to attend school and endure the discomfort, his condition worsened with the additional stressor of his father's abandonment. A family therapist at the mental health center determined after seeing him that he met the criteria for social phobia. A psychiatric evaluation also yielded a congruent diagnosis. His mother was only marginally able to be emotionally available to David because of her own grief. David needed the help of a team.

Intervention: The psychiatric provider placed David on an SSRI (selective serotonin reuptake inhibitor). Because of his mother's limited involvement in care and the potential for suicide in teens who are on an SSRI, David was placed on a twice-a-week visit schedule at the clinic. After a period of intense stabilization he attended weekly individual therapy, monthly group therapy, and monthly medication management. Over a period of two to three months he increased his school attendance, passed his classes, and developed a small peer group at school.

Resources. An overview of social phobia and research regarding the disorder in children and teens can be found at www2.massgeneral.org/schoolpsychiatry/info_socialphobia.asp. A compilation of prevalence data can be found at www.nimh.nih.gov/statistics/1SOC_CHILD.shtml. Teens themselves can find a relatable resource provided by the Nemours Foundation (1995–2012) at kidshealth.org/teen/your_mind/mental_health/social_phobia.html. A Canadian organization that helps families understand anxiety has a very practical and clinically appropriate management guide for parents of children with social phobia (AnxietyBC, 2007–2012). That resource can be found at www.anxietybc.com/sites/default/files/hmsocial.pdf.

Anorexia nervosa

Eating disorders are becoming of more concern not just because of their increased prevalence in teens, but also because of the potential for suicide. Eating disorders are often comorbid with other psychiatric conditions. The prevalence of anorexia nervosa in American youth is 0.3% (Swanson et al., 2011).

Amber is a 12-year-old Caucasian female of upper middle class background brought in to a mental health clinic by her parents. She refuses to eat. Although thin she is not emaciated; she is estimated to be 15% below ideal body weight for her height. Because she did not seem emaciated or gaunt her parents thought she was going through a "phase" but her behavior persisted. Her parents say that over the past six months she has been eating less and less. She plays with her food at the table or retires to her room to eat alone. She is very active, involved in sports, and aims to be a cheerleader in high school. Amber gets excellent grades, is well behaved, and very social. Amber's teachers have very positive regard for her. Physically she has met all developmental milestones. Noticeably, she does have lanugo and very thin hair. In discussing Amber's recent life stressors, her parents admit that about 6 months ago they were experiencing severe marital issues resulting in a brief separation. The separation ended because of their concern about Amber's issues with food. They initially tried to cajole and persuade Amber to eat; when that failed they attempted a firm approach and hoped to be able to force her to eat. Being unsuccessful with that strategy also they brought her in to the mental health center.

Impression. Amber's symptoms are consistent with an eating disorder. The presence of thinning hair and lanugo are symptoms of anorexia. An identifiable stressor is present. It is not uncommon for family discord, particularly between the parents of a child, to result in child distress. In Amber's case it appears that she exerted control over her eating when family functioning seemed out of her control.

Interventions. Medical intervention was necessary with regard to medication as well as general health status monitoring. A medication that helped reduce the core anxiety that Amber was experiencing was helpful. As in the case of administration of most drugs that treat anxiety or mood in teens, Amber's suicide potential was monitored once the medication was started. Regular lab work was necessary to make sure that Amber did not incur a severe electrolyte imbalance that could have precipitated a potentially fatal health crisis. Individual therapy was necessary for Amber, but it should be noted that family therapy was a significant part of her treatment as well. Her family therapist also focused on couples' therapy for Amber's parents. Management of their issues would be necessary to reduce Amber's anxiety. The treatment team included a nutrition consultant as well. Over time Amber was able to increase her food intake. The more she talked about her anxiety and sadness in therapy, the more she was able to relinquish some of the obsessive control she felt over food. Although Amber's progress was evident in the first six months of treatment, it was clear that she might need less intense but regular work over many years for her to experience remission.

Resources. For general information on eating disorders including anorexia nervosa information please visit the National Institutes of Health (2012) at the following web site: www.nimh.nih.gov/health/publications/eating-disorders/complete-index.shtml. A summary of research articles on the treatment of eating disorders may benefit family members. You can direct them to www .eating-disorder-resources.com/category/eating-disorder-articles/eating-disord er-treatment/.

Major depressive disorder

According to Merikangas et al. (2010) the prevalence of major depressive disorder in teens aged 13–18 is 11.2%. Although depression in children and teens can have symptoms that are similar to symptoms in adults, it should be noted that often there are slight differences with regard to both the number of symptoms and the duration of symptoms required for diagnosis. Additionally adolescent males may display more aggression and irritability than sadness.

> *Aaron is a 15-year-old African American male who is in a single parent household. His father is currently raising him as his mother abruptly left home six months ago. His 17-year-old sister and grandmother are also part of their household. His sister is a strong person who has achieved good grades and is highly responsible. She cares about Aaron and pressures him to behave well and to study hard. She encourages him to "get over" his current "funk." Aaron has been isolating himself from others and does not have friends with whom he spends time. He is withdrawn from his family too. Although he says school is important to him he has been truant and is failing two classes. Although uncharacteristic of him, he has gotten into two fights at school, primarily nonphysical. Both his eating patterns and his sleep have been erratic. His father caught him drinking after Aaron lied about taking his father's missing beer. Aaron confided in a school counselor that he was being bullied at school. He also told her that for the past week at least he has felt sad and angry. On her recommendation, Aaron was taken to his primary care doctor who referred him to the counseling center.*

Impression. Given the longer-than-one-week duration of sadness, anger, isolating behavior, appetite, and sleep changes, Aaron was evaluated for major depressive disorder. He met the criteria for the disorder. It appears that Aaron was attempting to forget his sadness by self-medicating with alcohol, which only made his depressive symptoms worse. Although his sister is supportive of him personally it seemed that the pressure to perform created some feelings of guilt or worthlessness in Aaron. A multidisciplinary approach to treatment was chosen.

Intervention. Aaron was first assessed by an individual therapist who assisted him in addressing his drinking behaviors. A substance abuse evaluation was conducted. Because Aaron was not addicted to alcohol, developing a plan for abstinence was possible with the help of Aaron's father. Aaron's individual therapist also assessed him for the potential of suicide. Aaron denied suicidality, and the medical provider was able to initiate treatment with an antidepressant. At the initiation of the antidepressant Aaron's entire family was educated on suicidality and assisted in monitoring Aaron for any surge of symptoms. Aaron's therapist also conducted family therapy to help the entire family grieve the loss of Aaron's mother and learn positive coping mechanisms and communication strategies that would strengthen their relationships with each other. Aaron's nurse from his primary care provider's office stayed involved in Aaron's process and scheduled him for a complete physical with his primary care provider so that any other physical contributors to Aaron's depressed mood could be ruled out. She helped Aaron develop a lifestyle plan that would ensure improvement in his eating and sleeping patterns. Aaron's therapist and nurse talked often and kept his treatment plan updated with the interventions occurring at both treatment venues. In individual therapy Aaron was able to discuss the bullying he experienced at school; he confessed that he felt that the bullying was racially driven. Aaron was successfully able to process issues of racism and low self-esteem in therapy. As Aaron became physically and mentally healthier at home, his therapist was able to work with Aaron's school to ensure a seamless treatment plan that would result in Aaron's success at school as well.

Resources. Teens such as Aaron may benefit from resources that they can access in language that is developmentally appropriate. Such a resource can be found at www.helpguide.org/mental/depression_teen_teenagers.htm. This site speaks to teens in a way that can decrease feelings of isolation and can validate their struggle. The NIMH (2012) fact sheet on teen depression may be validating for parents: www.nimh.nih.gov/health/topics/depression/depression-in-children-and-adolescents.shtml.

OTHER CONDITIONS

Within the confines of this chapter it is impossible to define and describe all the possible child conditions that can be encountered in nursing fieldwork. Here are some resources for some of those other conditions:

Attention deficit and hyperactivity disorder

The resources below are provided from both governmental (CDC, 2011) and private agencies (Children and Adults with Attention-Deficit/Hyperactivity Disorder, 2011).

1. www.cdc.gov/ncbddd/adhd/

2. www.help4adhd.org/en/about

Substance abuse

The national Substance Abuse and Mental Health Services Administration (2006, 2011) has created a web site (www.samhsa.gov/) through which parents can download brochures such as *Navigating the Teen Years: A Parent's Handbook for Raising Healthy Teens*. The web site has a publication section with a vast library of resources for professionals as well as lay individuals looking for treatment options.

CARING FOR THE CHILD WITH SPECIAL SOCIAL AND EMOTIONAL NEEDS

Post-traumatic stress disorder

The American Academy of Child and Adolescent Psychiatry (2011) provides useful information for medical providers and parents. Brochures can be found on their web site (www.aacap.org).

CONCLUSION

Social and emotional problems in children and teens must be addressed by nurses who are in a position to notice the behavior, systematically assess it, and bring together a team that can intervene to reduce its negative impact. In this chapter we have discussed clinical approaches to helping children and families and have also provided resources that various stakeholders may benefit from. Through consistent assessment and intervention it is possible to reduce the burden of illness on the child and family and set them up for future success.

REFERENCES

Achenbach, T. (2011). School age (ages 6–18) assessments. *Achenbach system of empirically based assessment.* Retrieved January 22, 2012, from http://aseba.org/schoolage.html

Achenbach, T.M., & Ruffle, T.M. (2000). The Child Behavior Checklist and related forms for assessing behavioral/emotional problems and competencies. *Pediatrics in Review*, 21(1), 265–271.

American Academy of Child and Adolescent Psychiatry. (2011). *Post Traumatic Stress Disorder: Facts for families.* Retrieved January 22, 2012, from http://aacap.org/page.ww?section=Facts for Families&name=Posttraumatic Stress Disorder (PTSD).

American Psychiatric Association. (2000). Diagnostic and statistical manual of mental disorders DSM-IV-TR. Washington, DC: Author.

AnxietyBC. (2007–2011). *Home management strategies for social anxiety disorder.* Retrieved January 22, 2012, from http://www.anxietybc.com/sites/default/files/hmsocial.pdf.

Bailey, A., Le Couteur, A., Gottesman, I., Bolton, P., Simonoff, E. Yuzda, E., & Rutter, M. (1995). Autism as a strongly genetic disorder: Evidence from a British twin study. *Psychological Medicine*, 25, 63–77.

Burstein, M., He, J.P., Kattan, G., Albano, A.M., Avenevoli, S., & Merikangas, K.R. (2011). Social phobia and subtypes in the national comorbidity survey – adolescent supplement: Prevalence, correlates, and comorbidity. *Journal of the American Academy of Child and Adolescent Psychiatry*, 50(9), 870–880.

Carson, V., & Trubowitz, J. (2006). Relevant Theories and Therapies for Nursing Practice. In E. Varcarolis, V. Benner & N. Shoemaker (Eds.), *Foundations of psychiatric and mental health nursing: A clinical approach* (pp. 15–33). St. Louis, MO: Saunders Elsevier.

Center for Epidemiological Studies Depression Scale for Children. (n.d.) *Bright Futures in Practice: Mental Health – Volume II, Toolkit*. Retrieved January 22, 2012, from http://www.brightfutures.org/mentalhealth/pdf/professionals/bridges/ces_dc.pdf

Centers for Disease Control and Prevention (CDC). (2012). *Autism Spectrum Disorders (ASDs)*. Retrieved November 18, 2012, from http://www.cdc.gov/ncbddd/autism/addm.html

Centers for Disease Control and Prevention (CDC). (2011). *Attention-Deficit/ Hyperactivity Disorder (ADHD)*. Retrieved January 22, 2012, from http://cdc.gov/ncbddd/adhd/.

Children and Adults with Attention-Deficit/Hyperactivity Disorder (CHADD). (2011). National Resource Center on ADHD: A Program of CHADD. Retrieved November 18, 2012, from http://help4adhd.org/.

Colson, C. (2006). Disorders of children and adolescents. In E. Varcarolis, V. Benner, & N. Shoemaker (Eds.), *Foundations of psychiatric and mental health nursing: A clinical approach* (pp. 634–657). St. Louis, MO: Saunders Elsevier.

Conners, C.K. (2004–2012). *Conners 3rd edition*. Retrieved January 22, 2012, from http://www.mhs.com/product.aspx?gr=cli&prod=conners3&id=overview

Eckendrode, J., Zielinski, D., Smith, E., Marcynyszyn, L.A., Henderson, C.R., & Kitzman, H. (2001). Child maltreatment and the early onset of problem behaviors: Can a program of nurse home visitation break the link? *Development and Psychopathology*, *13*, 873–890.

Hart, J., Gunnar, M., & Cicchetti, D. (1995). Salivary cortisol in maltreated children: Evidence of relations between neuroendocrine activity and social competence. *Development and Psychopathology*, *7*, 11–26.

Kessler, R.C., Berglund, P., Jin, R., et al. (2005). Lifetime prevalence and age-of-onset distributions of DSM-IV disorders in the National Comorbidity Survey Replication, *Archives of General Psychiatry*, *62*, 593–602.

Lombroso, P.J., Pauls, D.L., & Leckman, J.F. (1994). Genetic mechanisms in childhood psychiatric disorders. *Journal of the American Academy of Child and Adolescent Psychiatry*, *33*, 921–938.

Mash, E.J., & Dozois, D.J.A. (2003). Child psychopathology: A developmental-systems perspective. In E. Mash & R. Barkley (Eds.), *Child psychopathology* (2nd ed.)(pp. 3–71). New York, NY: Guilford Press.

Massachusetts General Hospital, School Psychiatry Program and MADI Resource Center. (2010). *For clinicians*. Retrieved November 18, 2012, from http://www2.massgeneral.org/schoolpsychiatry/for_clinicians.asp

McConaughy, S. (2005). *Clinical interviews for children and adolescents: Assessment to intervention*. New York, NY: Guilford Press.

Merikangas, K.R., He, J., Burstein, M., et al. (2010). Lifetime prevalence of mental disorders in U.S. adolescents: Results from the national comorbidity study – adolescent supplement (NCS-A). *Journal of the American Academy of Child and Adolescent Psychiatry*, *49*(10), 980–989.

Mitchell, S.A., & Black, M.J. (1995). *Freud and beyond: A history of modern psychoanalytic thought*. New York, NY: Basic Books.

Morrison, J., & Anders, T.E. (2001). *Interviewing children and adolescents: Skills and strategies for effective DSM-IV diagnosis*. New York, NY: The Guilford Press.

National Institutes of Mental Health. (2012a). *Depression in children and adolescents*. Retrieved January 22, 2012, from http://www.nimh.nih.gov/health/topics/depression/depression-in-children-and-adolescents.shtml.

National Institutes of Mental Health. (2012b). *Eating disorders.* Retrieved January 22, 2012, from http://www.nimh.nih.gov/health/publications/eating-disorders/complete -index.shtml.

Sadock, B.J., & Sadock, V.A. (2007). *Kaplan & Sadock's synopsis of psychiatry* (10th ed.). Philadelphia, PA: Lippincott Williams & Wilkins.

Substance Abuse and Mental Health Services Administration. (2011). *Prevention of substance abuse and mental illness.* Retrieved January 22, 2012, from http://www .samhsa.gov/prevention/.

Substance Abuse and Mental Health Services Administration. (2006). *Navigating the Teen Years: A Parents Handbook for Raising Healthy Teens.* http://store.samhsa.gov/ product/Navigating-the-Teen-Years-A-Parent-s-Handbook-for-Raising-Healthy-Tee ns/PHD1127

Swanson, S.A., Crow, S.J., Grange, D.L., et al. (2011). Prevalence and correlates of eating disorders in adolescents: Results from the National Comorbidity Survey Replication Adolescent Supplement. *Archives of General Psychiatry* (online March 7, 2011).

Taffel, R. (2005). *Breaking through to teens: Psychotherapy for the new adolescence.* New York, NY: Guilford Press.

The Nemours Foundation. (1995–2012). Social Phobia. *Teens Health from Nemours: For Teens.* Retrieved January 22, 2012, from http://kidshealth.org/teen/ your_mind/mental_health/social_phobia.html

Thomas, A., Chess, S., & Birch, H.G. (1965). *Your child is a person: A psychological approach to childhood without guilt.* New York, NY: Viking Press.

Varcarolis, E.M.(2006). Assessment strategies and the nursing process. In E. Varcarolis, V. Benner, & N. Shoemaker (Eds.), *Foundations of psychiatric and mental health nursing: A clinical approach* (pp. 138–154). St. Louis, MO: Saunders Elsevier.

Yeh, M., Hough, R.L., McCabe, K., Lau, A. & Garland, A. (2004). Parental beliefs about causes of child problems: Exploring racial/ethnic patterns. *Journal of the American Academy of Child and Adolescent Psychiatry, 43*(5), 605–612.

CARING FOR THE CHILD WITH
SPECIAL SOCIAL AND EMOTIONAL
NEEDS

CHAPTER 7
LEGAL AND REGULATORY ISSUES

Ginny Wacker Guido

Caring for Children with Special Healthcare Needs and Their Families: A Handbook for Healthcare Professionals, First Edition. Edited by Linda L. Eddy.
© 2013 John Wiley & Sons, Inc. Published 2013 by John Wiley & Sons, Inc.

INTRODUCTION

Individuals with disabilities comprise the nation's largest minority group, with 30.7% of the total national population experiencing some level of disability (US Census Bureau, 2008). The number of Children with disabilities is more difficult to determine, though the US Census Bureau estimated that approximately 20% of children ages 3–21 in 2005 had some level of disability.

One of the difficulties in determining the number of individuals with disabilities is that there is no single universal definition of the term "disability," either in federal law or in research on disability and disability services. For example, the Americans with Disabilities Act (ADA) of 1990 defined "disability" as "a physical or mental impairment that substantially limits one or more of the major life activities". Sometimes the definition is more restrictive, such as in the case of developmental disabilities, which affect approximately 1 of every 6 children 18 and younger (Centers for Disease Control, 2011). Such developmental disabilities are defined as chronic conditions that interfere with major life activities such as language, mobility, learning, self-help, and independent living. For the purposes of this chapter, children with disabilities are defined as those "having mental retardation, a hearing impairment (including deafness), a speech or language impairment, a visual impairment (including blindness), a serious emotional disturbance . . . an orthopedic impairment, autism, traumatic brain injury, other health impairment, a specific learning disability, deaf-blindness, or multiple disabilities, and who, by reason thereof, needs special education and related services" (Individuals with Disabilities Educational Act, 2004).

However disability is defined, education for all, frequently termed "inclusive education," should be the ultimate goal. The international policy agenda has proposed as a mandate Education for All (EFA), first adopted in March 1990. Participants from 155 countries and representatives of 160 government and nongovernmental agencies met for a world conference, adopting a world declaration that reaffirmed education as a basic human fundamental right. Interestingly, what is meant by *all* seems to be elusive. A subsequent report on EFA global monitoring mentions no progress toward inclusive education for children and youth with disabilities (Peters, 2007; United Nations Educational, Scientific, & Cultural Organization, 2004).

Assumptions that are inherent in inclusive education for those abled and disabled and thus in EFA include:

1. All students come to school with diverse needs and abilities, so no students are fundamentally different.

2. It is the responsibility of the general education system to be responsive to all students.

3. A responsive general education system provides high expectations and standards, quality academic curriculum and instruction that are flexible and relevant, an accessible environment, and teachers who are well prepared to address the educational needs of all students.

4. Progress in general education is a process evidenced by schools and communities working together to create citizens for an inclusive society who are educated to enjoy the full benefits, rights, and experiences of societal life. (Peters, 2007, p. 99)

CHILDREN WITH DISABILITIES AND THE LAW

In the United States, several laws protect the rights children with disabilities have in their educational pursuits. Some of these laws were enacted prior to the EFA mandate, but all model themselves on these four assumptions. Perhaps the law that is the best known is the Individuals with Disabilities Educational Act (IDEA) (2004).

Individuals with Disabilities Educational Act

The IDEA is a federal law governing how states and public agencies provide early intervention, special education, and related services to children with disabilities. The IDEA (2004) addresses the educational needs of children from birth to age 21, preparing these children for further education, employment, and independent living.

The IDEA is an example of "spending clause" legislation and is applicable only to the states and their local educational agencies that accept federal funding under this piece of legislation. Acceptance of IDEA funding makes public school districts responsible for identifying all students with disabilities in their district, regardless of whether they are attending public schools, as the law notes that private schools may not have the funding for providing accommodations under the Act. At present, all states have accepted funding under the IDEA.

The US education system has a long history of severely neglecting the needs of students with physical, mental, and learning disabilities. Until the enactment of the Education for All Handicapped Children Act (P.L. 94-142) in 1975, later codified as the IDEA, US public schools educated only one in five children with disabilities, leaving over one million children with disabilities having no access to public school systems, or segregating over three million students with disabilities to schools where they received little or no effective instruction (US Department of Education, n.d.; National Council on Disability, 2000).

The IDEA came about from federal case law holding that deprivation of free public education to children with disabilities constituted a deprivation of due process. Since its original enactment, the IDEA has been amended several times, most recently in December 2004. Key provisions of the IDEA include an individualized education program, free appropriate public education, provision of the least restrictive environment, provision of related services, and procedural safeguards. Additionally, there are also provisions for the discipline of children with disabilities.

Perhaps the best-known provision is the individualized education program (IEP). Viewed as the cornerstone of the child's educational program, the IEP specifies how and how often services are to be provided, describes the student's current levels of performance, indicates how the student's disabilities affect academic performance, and specifies modifications and accommodations to be provided to the student.

The IEP, designed to meet the student's unique education needs, mandates that these educational services and accommodations be provided in the least restrictive environment possible. This latter provision has been codified as "to the maximum extent appropriate, children with disabilities including children in public or private institutions or care facilities, are educated with children who are nondisabled" (IDEA, 2004, section 1412, 612(a)(5)). Any special classes, separate schooling, or the removal of children with disabilities from a regular educational environment is allowable only if the nature or severity of the disability is such that education in regular classrooms with the use of supplementary aids and services cannot be accomplished satisfactorily.

The concept that parent and family involvement and engagement improve student outcomes has particular implications for parents of children with IEPs (Underwood, 2010). Parent and family involvement and engagement in education are critical as strategies for supporting higher achievement for all school populations, with perhaps greater emphasis for children with disabilities as these joint conferences allow for more in-depth development of IEPs for the child's unique educational needs (Lee-Tarver, 2007). These authors concluded that the majority of teachers reported that all aspects of the IEP process was a team process and that valuable information was gained through the collaboration among teachers, counselors, and parents and family members.

Similar to the IEP, for children from birth to 3 years, the Individualized Family Service Plan (IFSP) assures that needed early intervention services are provided to children with disabilities. Inclusive preschool programs that serve these children and their facilities are generally Head Start and some university-affiliated programs (Peterson et al., 2004), though at least one research study (DeVore & Russell, 2007) concluded that programs in small rural communities could be equally effective in developing such inclusive programs. To be effective, these programs must include three dimensions: a family-centered orientation, natural and inclusive learning environments, and a collaborative team process (Bruder, 2010).

To further ensure that children with disabilities receive needed educational opportunities, the IDEA also has a provision entitled "Related Services." Such services may include transportation; services required to assist a child with a disability benefit from special education, including speech-pathology and audiology services; psychological services; physical and occupational therapy; music therapy; therapeutic recreation; counseling services; and medical services for diagnostic or evaluative purposes. This section has been expanded to include school health services, social work services in schools, and parent counseling and training (IDEA, 2004, section 1401(26)(A)).

The free appropriate public education (FAPE) provision means that the educational program is individualized to a specific child and designed to meet that child's unique educational needs, and it is from this program that the child receives educational benefits. The IDEA has further specified that the educational program provides access to the general curriculum that advances these children for further education, employment, and independent living. Safeguards to assure that children with disabilities receive a FAPE include giving multiple rights to the parents of these children. Some of the parental rights are the right to (a) review all educational records, (b) be equal partners on the IEP team, (c) participate in all aspects of planning their child's education, (d) file complaints to the state educational agency, (e) request medication or a due process hearing, (f) present an alternative IEP and their witnesses to support their case, and (g) engage in Alternative Dispute Resolution (ADR) hearings and appeal from the results of those hearings.

Finally, the IDEA provides guidance for the discipline of children with disabilities. Specifically, the disability must be taken into account when disciplinary actions are taken. The IDEA focuses on the need to use appropriate behavioral interventions and functional behavioral assessments in determining the best educational setting for the student with disabilities and others in the classroom. Note, though, that a student who brings a weapon to a school or school function, or possesses, uses, or sells illegal drugs or controlled substances at school or a school function, or causes serious bodily injury to another person, may be placed in an interim alternate educational setting for up to 45 days. This allows the student to continue to receive educational services while the IEP team determines appropriate actions and/or placement for the student.

LEGAL AND REGULATORY ISSUES

No Child Left Behind Act

The No Child Left Behind Act of 2001 (NCLB) is the most recent version of the Elementary and Secondary Education Act (ESEA), the nation's major federal law related to education in prekindergarten through high school. First passed in 1965, the ESEA was part of the nation's war on poverty with the centerpiece Title 1, a provision designed to improve achievement among the nation's poor and disadvantaged students. The full title of the NCLB Act aptly begins to define its purpose: An act to close the achievement gap with accountability, flexibility, and choice, so that no child is left behind (P.L. 107-110). The NCLB Act supports standards-based education, which is based on the premise that setting high standards and establishing measurable goals will result in improvement in education scores for individual students. States receiving federal funding for schools are required to develop assessments in basic skills to be administered to all students in selected grades. The Act does not set a national achievement standard, but allows the individual states to set their standard.

The impetus behind the NCLB legislation was the argument that local governments were not mandating sufficiently high standards to assure that schools were meeting their objectives, and that schools were particularly lax in meeting the educational needs of traditionally underserved groups of children, such as low-income and minority students. Supporters of the Act argued that local governments had failed students in general, and that federal intervention was needed to prevent teachers from teaching outside their expertise or maintaining an attitude of complacency in light of poor student performance. By focusing on the basic skills of reading, writing, and mathematics, the NCLB Act seeks to assure that life skills for all students, not just those college-bound or affluent, are at or are progressing toward proficiency.

Supporters of the Act noted that one of the most positive points of the legislation is the increased accountability required by schools and instructors. Schools are required to pass yearly tests that judge the difference in improvement that the students have made during the fiscal year. These yearly standardized tests are the deciding factor in whether the schools are meeting the standards in regard to student outcomes. If improvements cannot be shown through the students' test results, the schools face decreased federal funding in subsequent fiscal years.

To begin to assure that students were taught by competent instructors, the Act mandates minimal qualifications for teachers, including (a) a bachelor's degree; (b) full state competency, credentialing, or licensure; and (c) periodic demonstration of continued competency. The NCLB Act further mandates that every state (a) measure the extent to which all students have highly qualified teachers, particularly minority and disadvantaged students; (b) implement plans to assure continuing teacher competency; and (c) publicly report plans and measure progress on meeting teacher quality goals.

Under the NCLB, states must make available every reasonable adaptation and accommodation for students with disabilities. One means of accommodating the educational needs of children with disabilities is to implement co-teaching models rather than the more traditional model of a single instructor. The co-teaching model is designed to be more inclusive of disabled students in regular classroom settings as the model combines a general education instructor with a special education instructor. Both instructors are responsible for teaching all of the students in the classroom. Advantages of this co-teaching model are that it increases instructional opportunities for students and enhances the participation and performance of students with disabilities (Nichols, Dowdy, & Nichols, 2010). Further advantages include that all students receive the attention of two instructors, who offer a more enriched curriculum than would be afforded by a single instructor.

The NCLB legislation also expects that the vast majority of students with disabilities will participate in the same assessment tests that all other students take. Unfortunately, the major disadvantage of the co-teaching model concerned these standardized tests. Specifically, there was increased pressure to move students quickly through material that would be evaluated on standardized tests. The students who were shown to be least able to achieve the needed leaning were those with learning disabilities (Mastropieri et al., 2005).

For standardized tests, reasonable adaptation and accommodations are generally grouped into four categories: (a) presentation; (b) response; (c) timing/scheduling; or (d) setting. Thus, the testing may be in the form of allowing extra breaks during the test, using larger bubbles on answer sheets, using computer rather than handwritten testing methodologies, allowing additional time to complete the test, reading the test to the child, taking the test in a separate room, or perhaps employing a Braille edition of the test for students who are vision-impaired. The academic content, though, remains unchanged and students with disabilities participate in the same assessments that all students take.

Because not all children with disabilities have the cognitive ability to take standardized tests, NCLB allows an alternate assessment based on alternate achievement standards. These alternate assessment tests measure the student's progress on state grade-level content standards, but at a reduced breath, depth, or complexity, and the results are judged against a different definition of proficiency than the regular assessment. The decision regarding whether a specific student will participate in an alternate assessment-based test is made by the IEP team. Thus, there is some overlap between the IDEA and NCLB.

In June 2011, Education Secretary Arne Duncan announced that if Congress fails to take action to rewrite the NCLB legislation, he will initiate steps to ease some of the more punitive aspects of the current law (Banchero & Meckler, 2011). Currently the law requires states to show student proficiency in mathematics and reading through the administration of standardized tests. Duncan has projected that by March 2012, the vast majority of public schools will miss their ever-increasing target pass rates on these tests, thus opening states to possible sanctions, such as requirements mandating specialized tutoring or allowing students to transfer to other schools. Secretary Duncan proposed that states should be allowed to adopt alternate efforts of accountability, such as linking teacher evaluations to student achievements, expanding charter schools, and overhauling the lowest-performing schools. Whatever the outcome, the goal should be comprehensive educational reform for all children (Brown, 2011). In early August 2011 (Turner, 2011), it was announced that states could apply for waivers from the program. In return, states granted waivers would be required to implement tougher evaluation systems for instructors and tackle the achievement gap for minority and disadvantage children.

Americans with Disabilities Act of 1990

The American with Disabilities Act of 1990 (ADA) was enacted to assure that individuals with disabilities, including children, have the same access to programs, activities, and services as their nondisabled peers. Though not specific to education, the ADA must also be considered when reviewing the legal rights of children with disabilities.

The ADA was amended in November 2008, in what is now known as the Americans with Disabilities Amended Act (ADAA). Portions of the amended act that relate to disabled students' education include the eligibility requirements. The amended act expanded the eligibility for individual students under section 504 of the Rehabilitation Act of 1973 and reinforced the regulatory overlap for students who have IEPs under the IDEA Act of 2004. Primarily, the expanded coverage under the ADAA pertains to the second and third eligibility criteria for disability: the mental or physical impairment must limit a major life activity to a substantial extent.

Regarding major life events, the ADAA expanded the major life event beyond walking, seeing, hearing, and learning to include newly codified learning-related impairments such as concentrating, reading, and thinking. The criterion of "to a substantial extent" was broadened to include episodic conditions as well as conditions in remission, so that a student may be considered eligible under the ADAA for episodic conditions during their active state, such as anaphylactic effects of severe food allergies or episodes of severe hypoglycemia or hyperglycemia in diabetic children.

Though these new interpretive standards raise questions as to eligibility and resulting entitlements for school-age children, the overall effect of this amended act is the expansion of the number and range of students eligible under section 504. Educators need to consider carefully how these new standards will result in obligations to eligible students and whether these newly eligible students will automatically require section 504 plans with their IEPs.

ETHICAL ISSUES IN CARING FOR CHILDREN WITH DISABILTIES

Multiple ethical principles and values drive the care for children with disabilities. Society has an obligation to ensure that children can reach and maintain their full potential and an acceptable quality of life, whatever that individual potential may be. Disabled children have the human right to be included in their local communities and to receive the same quality education as their nondisabled peers. These rights are rooted in four basic ethical principles: respect for autonomy; beneficence; nonmaleficence; and justice (Beauchamp & Childress, 2008).

The respect-for-autonomy principle clearly supports the need to assure the adequate education of the disabled child to the full extent of the individual child's capabilities. Children with disabilities have the right to free and appropriate education in the most inclusive settings possible, using reasonable accommodations as needed, and being allowed, as they are able, to take part in activities and programs that are available to nondisabled peers. These expectations are at the foundation of the IDEA legislation, noting that Act prepares the child for future education, employment, and independent living to the full extent possible.

Embedded in the respect for autonomy are the remaining principles of beneficence, nonmaleficence, and justice. Each of these principles further support the obligations of the educational system to provide for the good of the child with disabilities, in a manner that prevents harm from occurring, and assuring that these children have as equitable assess to educational opportunities as their nondisabled peers.

Perhaps a deeper understanding of the ethics that underlie the whole of the educational system in general and the quality of education for disabled children in specific is the ethic of caring. Though often characterized as feminine because the ethical orientation seems to arise more naturally from women's experiences rather than men's experiences, this ethical orientation is more naturally centered on an understanding of the individual as an interdependent, relational being, and emphasizes the importance of human relationships. Care ethics notes that human beings are essentially dependent on one another; for example, children are dependent upon their parents or parent surrogates for their well-being. This creates a reciprocal responsibility in parents or parent surrogates to care for their children and provide the most appropriate care possible. One could argue that this translates to the whole of the educational system, creating the responsibility of educators to provide appropriate and quality educational opportunities for all children, the disabled as well as the nondisabled. Certainly, the ethics of caring appropriately underlie both the IDEA and the ADAA.

The NCLB legislation, however, raises multiple ethical concerns, primarily because of its basic components. The four major components of this legislation are: enhanced accountability, additional freedoms for states and individual communities, educational methodologies that are well-founded, and additional choices for parents. Imbedded in these components are that educational programs most notably enhance opportunities for two specific portions of the population: minorities and the poor. This preference for these two populations raises the ethical challenges of fairness, social justice, and equality. Educators should expect that all students demonstrate proficiency, and should demand that all students work to their full capacity, which may or may not be achieved through success on standardized test scores. This expectation raises the issue of whether the law has achieved its accountability component. An alternate way of addressing this query is through the foundation of social justice. This aspect will best be considered when it is evident that the NCLB legislation treats all individuals in a fair and just manner.

At present, states are implementing the NCLB law as deemed appropriate for their populations, which means that the law is interpreted and implemented differently in various states. Thus, students may be treated differently as they move from one state to another state. These interpretations may also mean that students are selectively excluded or included while other groups receive alternate educational standards. For example, school officials may focus on students who have not yet achieved proficiency while selectively disregarding the needs of those students who exceed a specific standard or are so far below the standard that achievement is viewed as unobtainable.

These principles are further impacted by the fact that a single standard does not simultaneously challenge students at all levels, thus violating the principle of equity (Hoff & Olsen, 2006). They argued that this "one size fits all" concept should not apply to education. Rothstein, Jacobsen, and Wilder (2006) further noted that for the law to be equitable it must address the achievement gap within groups of students, including within groups of nonwhites and groups of whites, not between groups of nonwhites and whites. This is further supported by Sack (2007), who believed the law will never achieve its intent as it disregards the root causes of the educational achievement gap as seen in American education today.

Ethics are the standards that should be considered when implementing decisions that affect the education of children. Education officials have an obligation to support the interests of all students, the disabled as well as the nondisabled, and those with greater educational requirements. Because of the ethical challenges associated with the NCLB legislation, there needs to be continued dialogue on how to assure that the principles of fairness, social justice, and equality are implemented.

LAWS AFFECTING THE EDUCATION OF DISABLED CHILDREN AND THE HEALTHCARE SYSTEM

School nurses play an essential role in the seamless provision of comprehensive healthcare services. Increasingly, more and more children entering school systems have chronic health conditions and disabilities that require expert management during the school day. As defined by the National Association of School Nurses (1999), school nursing is:

> *A specialized practice of professional nursing that advances the well-being, academic success, and lifelong achievement of students. To that end, school nurses facilitate positive student responses to normal development; promote health and safety; intervene with actual and potential health problems; provide case management services; and actively collaborate with others to build student and family capacity for adaptation, self-management, self-advocacy, and learning. (p. 1)*

Inherent in this definition are multiple roles that the school nurse fulfills, including: providing direct care to students for injuries, acute illness, and the long-term management of students with special healthcare needs; providing leadership for the provision of appropriate health services; and serving as the liaison between school officials, family members, healthcare professionals, and the community. These roles directly relate to the education of children with disabilities.

The IDEA grants to eligible children with disabilities the right to receive free appropriate public education in the least restrictive settings possible. Access for these children is achieved through the provision of necessary healthcare, which may include the administration of oral and intravenous medications, catheterization, tracheostomy care, and gastrostomy feedings, among other care procedures. To assure that providing this care is accomplished safely and competently, the role of the school nurse has been greatly expanded in recent years.

Under both the IDEA and the NCLB legislation, children with disabilities are entitled to support services at school. These are generally known as "related" services. In the early enactment of the IDEA, there was no specific requirement as to whom would provide these related services, though the Congressional Record noted that there could be situations where a licensed registered nurse should be part of the IEP team (Schwab, Gelfman, & Cohn, 2001). Prior to 1999, many jurisdictions continued to rely on multidisciplinary teams in the development and the implementation of students' IEPs or IFSPs. This resulted in the delivery of healthcare services that were either not included or were provided in an improper manner, performed by individuals who lacked the necessary education and supervision to provide such services.

This change in 1999 came about as a result of a US Supreme Court ruling in the case of *Cedar Rapids Community School District v. Garret F.* (generally referred to as *Garret F.*). The case involved a wheelchair-bound and ventilator-dependent schoolchild who required, in part, a responsible individual nearby to attend to his physical needs during the school day. The Community School District refused to accept financial responsibility for the services that Garret required, believing that it was not legally obligated to provide one-to-one nursing care. The requested services in this case were supporting services because the child could not attend school without them. Nor were the required services medical services, because they could competently be delivered by registered nurses educated in the care of ventilator-dependent children.

The Supreme Court specifically addressed the section of the IDEA that mandates that its purpose is to "assure all children with disabilities have available to them . . . a free and appropriate public education which emphasizes special education and related services designed to meet their unique needs" (IDEA, 1995, section 1400(c)). Thus, the holding of the court was that these services were the obligation of the school district, as these services were needed by Garret to be assisted to "meaningfully access public school" within the meaning of the IDEA.

This ruling has impacted school districts in multiple ways. First, it made clear the concept that school districts were financially responsible for providing school nursing services when such supportive services are necessary in order for students with disabilities to be able to access and benefit from the educational programs. Two, it made very clear that these supporting nursing services could include any level of service on a continuum, from direct to indirect nursing care one hour per week, a nurse on site at all times, or one-to-one nursing care throughout the entire school day. Three, nursing as a vital part of the

LEGAL AND REGULATORY ISSUES

multidisciplinary team that develops and implements the IEP or the IFSP was fully recognized. Perhaps this last impact of the ruling is the most significant from the perspective of students with disabilities. Parents of children with disabilities should insist that their child's IEP or ISFP include necessary nursing services as a part of the form. Such an inclusion further ensures that their child will receive the necessary services needed to assure that the child receives the best educational opportunities available.

CONCLUSION

Multiple strides have been made during the last few decades to begin to assure that children with disabilities have the same educational opportunities that are available to those without disabilities. The laws that have been enacted since the mid-1960s have continued to address issues that relate to the educational opportunities that these children may receive. This chapter has focused on the successes and continuing challenges that these laws have addressed as well as what still must be addressed to truly ensure that all children receive at all grade levels the highest quality of education that can be provided in the United States.

REFERENCES

Americans with Disabilities Act. (1990). 42 U.S.C. § 12102(2).

Beauchamp, T., & Childress, J.F. (2008). *Principles of biomedical ethics* (6th ed.). New York, NY: Oxford University Press.

Banchero, S., & Meckler, L. (2011, June 12). Duncan threatens to alter No Child Left Behind. *Wall Street Journal.* Retrieved from http://online.wsj.com/article/SB10001424052702304259304576378104116703210.html

Brown, C.G. (2011). Reauthorize, reauthorize, reauthorize No Child Left Behind. Retrieved from http://www.americanprogress.org/issues/2011/06/nclbwaivers.html

Bruder, M.B. (2010). Early childhood intervention: A promise to children and families for their future. *Exceptional Children, 76*(3), 339–355.

Cedar Rapids Community School District v. Garret F., 119 S. Ct. 992, (1999).

Centers for Disease Control.(2011). Developmental disabilities increasing in the United States. Atlanta GA: Author.

DeVore, S., & Russell, K. (2007). Early childhood education and care for children with disabilities: Facilitating inclusive practice. *Early Childhood Education Journal, 35*(2), 189–198.

Education for All Handicapped Children Act (1975) Public Law 94–142.

Hoff, D. & Olsen, D. (2006). Researchers ask whether NCLB's goals for proficiency are realistic. *Education Week, 26*(13), 8.

Individuals with Disabilities Act (1990). 20 U.S.C. §§ 1400 et seq.

Individuals with Disabilities Act (2004). 20 U.S.C. § 1412, 612(a)(5).

Lee-Tarver, A. (2007). Are individualized education plans a good thing? A survey of teachers' perceptions of the utility of IEPs in regular education settings. *Journal of Instructional Psychology*, *33*(4), 263–272.

Mastropieri, M., Scruggs, T., Graetz, J., et al. (2005). Case study in co-teaching in the content areas: Successes, failures, and challenges. *Intervention in School and Clinic*, *40*(5), 260–270.

National Association of School Nurses. (1999). *Definition of school nursing.* Silver Spring, MD: Author. Retrieved from www.nasn.org

National Council on Disability. (2000). Back to school on civil rights: Advancing the federal commitment to Leave No Child Behind. Washington DC: Author.

Nichols, J., Dowdy, A., & Nichols, C. (2010). *Education*, *130*(4), 647–651.

Peters, S.J. (2007). A historical analysis of international inclusive education policy and individuals with disabilities. *Journal of Disability Policy Studies*, *18*(2), 98–108.

Peterson, C., Wall, S., Raikes, H., et al. (2004). Early Head Start: Identifying and serving children with disabilities. *Topics in Early Childhood Special Education*, *24*(2), 76–88.

Rothstein, R., Jacobsen, R., & Wilder, T. (2006). Proficiency for all is an oxymoron. *Education Week*, *26*(13), 32–44.

Schwab, N., Gelfman, M., & Cohn, S. (2001). IDEA: Current issues in dispute. In N.C. Schwab & M. Gelfman (Eds.), *Legal issues in school health services: A resource for school administrators, school attorneys, and school nurses.* (pp. 399–418). North Branch, MN: Sunrise River Press.

Turner, D. (2011, August 9). States can get waivers on No Child tests. *The Columbian*, p. A2.

Underwood, K. (2010). Involving and engaging parents of children with IEPs. *Exceptionality Education International*, *20*(1), 18–36.

United Nations Educational, Scientific, and Cultural Organization. (2004). *EFA: The quality imperative.* Paris: Author.

US Census Bureau. (2008). Americans with disabilities 2005: Household economic studies. Washington, DC: Author.

US 34 Code of Federal Regulations, sections 300.304 through 300.311.

US Department of Education, Office of Special Education and Rehabilitation Services. (n.d.). *History: Twenty-five years of progress in educating children with disabilities through IDEA.* Washington, DC: Author.

LEGAL AND REGULATORY ISSUES

RESOURCES FOR PARENTS

Cortiella, C. (2006). NCLB and IDEA: What parents of students with disabilities need to know and do. Minneapolis: University of Minnesota, National Center on Educational Outcomes.

http://www2.ed.gov/about/offices/list/osers/osep/index.html Office of Special Education and Rehabilitative Services

http://www.nichcy.org/Pages/Home.aspx National Dissemination Center for Children with Disabilities

http://www.heath.gwu.edu/ Resource Center: Online Clearing House on Postsecondary Education for Individuals with Disabilities http://www.parentcenternetwork.org/national/aboutus.html Alliance: National Parent Technical Assistance Center

http://www.taalliance.org/resources/spanish.asp Alliance: Technical Assistance for Parent Centers (Spanish edition)

http://osepideasthatwork.org/parentkit/index.asp Tool Kit on Teaching and Assessing Students with Disabilities (written specifically for parents)

LEGAL AND REGULATORY ISSUES

CHAPTER 8
USE OF THEORIES TO GUIDE PRACTICE

Linda L. Eddy

Caring for Children with Special Healthcare Needs and Their Families: A Handbook for Healthcare Professionals, First Edition. Edited by Linda L. Eddy.
© 2013 John Wiley & Sons, Inc. Published 2013 by John Wiley & Sons, Inc.

Child healthcare in general, and care of children with disabilities in particular, is increasingly dependent on sound theoretical bases. This chapter outlines common individual and family theories that can help to structure our care of children and adolescents as well as provide guidance in accomplishing comprehensive family assessment and intervention. Individual theories include: (a) Erikson's stages of psychosocial development, and (b) Piaget's stages of cognitive development. Family theories include: (a) family life course perspective (developmental family theory), (b) family systems theory, and (c) various contextual theories. Examples of use of these theories when caring for children with a variety of special healthcare needs are offered. Brief, clinically useful theory-based individual and family assessment guidelines are also provided.

INDIVIDUAL THEORIES

Professionals caring for children generally have a good knowledge of child growth and development and just need to understand differences that may impact care of children with special healthcare needs. Additionally, although similarities may exist between children based on diagnosis or developmental level, it is important to remember that each child is unique.

Physical growth and development

The guiding principle here is the idea of pattern or trajectory. Children with special needs, whether physical, developmental, or both, grow and develop in a way that is more similar than different from children without special needs. In particular, their growth and development progresses in the same general pattern or order as that of a child without special needs, but the rate of growth and development may differ. Therefore, it is very important to have accurate information about the child's baseline growth and development. Standardized charts and assessment tools may not accurately represent the child with special needs, and only assessment of growth and development in relation to the baseline will provide a window into issues needing immediate attention.

Erikson's theory of psychosocial development

Erik Erikson believed that psychosocial development occurred in a series of stages that continue throughout the life span. Erikson believed that a sense of competence also motivated behaviors and actions. Each stage in Erikson's theory is concerned with becoming competent in an area of life (1968). If the stage is handled well, the person will feel a sense of mastery. If the stage is managed poorly, the person will emerge with a sense of inadequacy. In each stage, Erikson believes people experience a conflict that serves as a turning point in development. In Erikson's view, these conflicts are centered on either developing a psychological quality or failing to develop that quality. During these times, the potential for personal growth is high, but so is the potential for failure. For reference, each stage in this theory is outlined based on information from Erikson's seminal work *Childhood and Society* (1968), and an example is offered on application to children with special needs. Because this handbook is focused on care of children, only stages one through five will be examined. It is important to remember, however, that development continues throughout the life span.

Psychosocial Stage 1 – trust versus mistrust. The first stage of Erikson's theory of psychosocial development occurs between birth and one year of age and is the most fundamental stage in life (Erikson, 1963). Because an infant is utterly dependent, the development of trust is based on the dependability and quality of the child's caregivers. If a child successfully develops trust, he or she will feel safe and secure in the world. Caregivers who are inconsistent, emotionally unavailable, or rejecting contribute to feelings of mistrust in the children they care for. Failure to develop trust will result in fear in the child and a belief that the world is inconsistent and unpredictable.

Parents or caregivers of an infant with a disability that involves lack of social response, such as autism, might respond to the lack of social smile or other social cues by failing to meet the infant's need for nurturing, resulting in the infant's lack of trust in the world. This could happen well before autism or other global developmental delays are even diagnosed. Nurses and other pediatric healthcare providers can contribute to preventing this reciprocal downward spiral by ensuring that all parents have the necessary knowledge about the importance of bonding and attachment for maximizing the infant's emotional and social development.

Psychosocial Stage 2 – autonomy versus shame and doubt. The second stage of Erikson's theory of psychosocial development takes place during early childhood and is focused on children developing a greater sense of personal control. Like Freud, Erikson believed that toilet training was a vital part of this process. However, Erikson's reasoning was quite different than that of Freud's. Erikson believed that learning to control one's body functions leads to a feeling of control and a sense of independence. Other important events include gaining more control over food choices, toy preferences, and clothing selection. Children who successfully complete this stage feel secure and confident, whereas those who do not are left with a sense of inadequacy and self-doubt.

For a child with a special healthcare need that involves lack of mobility or bowel and bladder continence, such as spina bifida, the path to autonomy is different but no less important. The healthcare provider uses his or her understanding of the toddler's need for autonomy to structure the inpatient or outpatient environment to maximize the child's ability to influence that environment. Facilitating autonomy by encouraging each child to be as independent as possible is time-consuming for care providers, and extra time for caring for children with special healthcare needs has to be built into the professionals' caseloads. In the same way, healthcare professionals can help parents develop realistic schedules that allow for the extra time required by a child who is trying to master his or her environment.

Psychosocial Stage 3 – initiative versus guilt. During the preschool years, children begin to assert their power and control over the world through directing play and other social interaction. Children who are successful at this stage feel capable and able to lead others. Those who fail to acquire these skills are left with a sense of guilt, self-doubt, and lack of initiative.

Peer relationships are key in developing healthy social and emotional lives. Preschoolers with communication differences might have difficulty interacting with same-age peers. Speech and language pathologists, occupational therapists, and other members of the healthcare team can consult with early childhood educators about communication strategies necessary for young children with special needs to be included in peer groups. In the inpatient setting, members of the healthcare team need to include communication strategies used by each child in admission and ongoing assessments. For example, hospital admission of Aaron, a 4-year-old boy with intellectual disabilities and speech delays, must include a session with Aaron's family in which they teach the healthcare professionals about Aaron's communication board and how to understand his rudimentary sign language so that his healthcare team is able to communicate with him in this unfamiliar environment.

Psychosocial Stage 4 – industry versus inferiority. This stage covers the early school years from approximately age 5 to 11. Through social interactions, children begin to develop a sense of pride in their accomplishments and abilities. Children who are encouraged and commended by parents and teachers develop a feeling of competence and belief in their skills. Those who receive little or no encouragement from parents, teachers, or peers will doubt their ability to be successful.

Children with intellectual disabilities and other learning differences are at risk for developing a sense of inferiority if their progress is measured on the yardstick of the typically developing child. Because child development occurs across a similar pattern for most children, with differences that are more in rate rather than type of skill acquisition, healthcare providers need to teach parents and caregivers the importance of celebrating small steps in development. This may be more difficult for parents whose other children have progressed quickly or who have rigid expectations for their children, but if parents understand the importance of their praise and support in fostering children's belief in themselves, most parents adjust quickly to changed expectations.

Psychosocial Stage 5 – identity versus identity confusion. During adolescence, children are exploring their independence and developing a sense of self. Those who receive proper encouragement and reinforcement through personal exploration will emerge from this stage with a strong sense of self and a feeling of independence and control. Those who remain unsure of their beliefs and desires will feel insecure and confused about themselves and the future.

Independence and control might look different for children with special healthcare needs, but they are important factors in the healthy emotional development of all children. Many adolescents with physical disabilities that restrict independent mobility, such as cerebral palsy or muscular dystrophy, use assistive devices to enhance their independence. Encouraging these young adults to participate in adaptive sports or other activities where they can excel can result in a sense of mastery and control.

Piaget's theory of cognitive development

Like Erikson, Jean Piaget believed that development progressed along a continuum that was more similar than different for most children (Pontious, 1982; Richmond, 1971). Unlike Erikson, however, Piaget was more interested in the cognitive development of children than in their social and emotional growth.

According to Piaget, the way the child thinks, reasons, and uses language differs significantly in each of the following age groups: sensorimotor (birth to 2 years), preoperational (2 to 7 years), concrete operations or school-age (7 to 12 years), and formal operations, or adolescence and beyond (Richmond, 1971). Infants in the sensorimotor stage of development learn about the world through their senses and have very undeveloped thought and reasoning abilities. Emerging language is basically imitative, and therefore verbal explanations are of little use. Children in the preoperational stage see things from their own perspective, and thinking is literal and concrete. These young children also think in absolutes: something is either good or bad, right or wrong, etc. Preoperational children can focus on only one aspect of a situation or object, and can judge others' actions only in regard to their impact on him or her. School-age children in Piaget's concrete operations stage are capable of seeing the world more realistically and of seeing things from the viewpoint of others. They are becoming more flexible and relative in their thinking, and are able to appreciate more than one aspect of an object or situation. They reason deductively, by trial and error, and are beginning to be able to judge others' actions by their logical effect. Words now represent real objects or concepts, and the concrete operational child is able to use words to communicate and learn about the world. Although school-age children may have some understanding of past and future, these children still have difficulty with abstractions and with worlds that stand for things they have yet to experience (Pontious, 1982). Adolescents, in Piaget's formal operational stage, think and reason as do adults, although their actions and behaviors are not yet fully mature.

Healthcare team members can use this understanding of the way children think and reason to tailor their healthcare teaching for children with special healthcare needs and their families. To do this, however, we have to consider the child's or adolescent's developmental age rather than just his or her chronological age. Realistic expectations for children and their families demand that level of understanding of the nature of a particular child's thought, reasoning, and language abilities. For example, an 8-year-old child with a developmental age of 4 years (DQ = 0.5), even with understandable spoken language, would not be expected to understand that some shots hurt a lot while others do only a little. In the same way, an adolescent with a developmental age of 8 years would likely not understand the possible side effects of a medication that he or she is to take.

However, it is important to remember that development can occur unevenly for children with special healthcare needs, and healthcare team members need to guard against thinking that children with disabilities such as cerebral palsy are necessarily cognitively delayed in all areas, or even delayed at all. For example, although many children with severe physical disabilities are delayed in development of spatial abilities, a study by Rothman (1989) demonstrated that many of those physical disabilities did not interfere with cognitive development not dependent upon spatial concepts. When engaging in care planning and patient and family education, the healthcare team, parents, and caregivers need a comprehensive understanding of the child's cognitive function in order to target the child's strengths and challenges.

FAMILY THEORIES

Child healthcare is based on the understanding of family as client, and this conceptualization underscores the need to understand not only individual child development, but development of the family. Healthcare team members are often at a loss when it comes to meeting the needs of the family of a child with a special health need. A basic understanding of family development and family processes can help us meet these needs in a sensitive, respectful, and useful manner. Most theories used to understand what is happening in families are borrowed from other disciplines, such as social science and economics, but have been modified for use with families. One such theory is the family life course perspective, often called developmental family theory.

USE OF THEORIES TO
GUIDE PRACTICE

Table 8.1 Stages of Psychosocial and Cognitive Development

Age In years	Erikson's Conflicts Psychosocial	Piaget Cognitive
0–1	Trust vs. Mistrust	Sensorimotor
1–1 1/2	Autonomy vs. Shame	
1 1/2–2		
1–2		
2–4	Initiative vs. Guilt	Preoperational
4–5		
5–6	Industry vs. Inferiority	
6–7		
7–8		Concrete Operational
8–9		
9–10		
10–11		
11–12		Formal Operational
12-13	Identity vs.Identity Confusion	
13–20s		
20s–30s	Intimacy vs. Isolation	
30s–35		
35–40s		
40s–50s	Generativity vs. Stagnation	
50s–60s	Integrity vs. Despair	
60s–70s		
70s–80s		
Above 85		

Family life course perspective (developmental family theory)

Time influences relationships in several ways. The behavior of individuals in a family is in part a function of the individual's development as well as the level of development of other family members. The behavior of individuals in families is also a function of generational placement because of roles and expectations. Life experiences influence relationships. Family events and family transitions influence individuals and interactions. Historical time – events in the broader social context – influence roles and values. Individuals are influenced by social context. Social structures (racism, sexism, homophobia) influence individual development. Social structures change, and this change influences individuals and relationships. Individuals actively interact with social context and structure. This produces a reciprocal influence between families/individuals and social context via socially constructed meaning systems.

Although there has been criticism of this theory in that it is too determin-istic (in other words, there is concern about the ideas that behavior can be predicted, that there are a particular set of stages that all must follow, and that if certain conditions are met families will move through their family "career" successfully), the theory is useful in emphasizing the changing social nature of individuals and families over time. In our context, understanding that time influences relationships can help to explain why parents who have just been told about their child's diagnosis are often angry and may act out at the healthcare team. Now may not be the best time for complex anticipatory guidance for this family; waiting until the parents have time to adjust to this family transition will likely improve the provider-family relationship and render care more useful.

Systems theory

Key assumptions. A systems view looks at the world in terms of sets of integrated relations – in other words, in terms of how subsystems interact with each other (Whitchurch & Constantine, 1993). In family systems theory the focus is on these interactions rather than on the parts themselves. For example, the focus on the interconnectedness of families rather than their separateness helps professionals understand better how something affecting one member of a family (such as illness or disability) affects the entire family.

Basic systems terminology

- System: a goal-directed unit made up of interdependent, interacting parts

- Nonsummativity: the whole is greater than the sum of its parts

- Open system: a high level of interactivity with its environment

- Closed system: a low level of or interactivity with its environment

- Boundary: Point of contact between the system and its subsystems or suprasystems

- Differentiation: the capacity to grow and change

- Adaptation: the capacity to modify based on input

- Self-reflectivity: the capacity of human systems to "think about themselves"

The family systems approach regards the family, as a whole, as the client or as the unit of care, and emphasizes such factors as relationships and communication patterns rather than traits or symptoms in individual members. Having a child or adolescent with special healthcare needs affects the whole family and others outside the family who are integral to the healthy functioning of the family. Therefore, it makes sense to structure care for these families based on existing relationships and communication patterns, and to work with the families to strengthen these patterns and relationships. For example, in the case study of Mia introduced in Chapter 1, child and family outcomes would likely be improved by helping Mia's parents find ways of talking about their feelings regarding her diagnosis. Healthcare professionals can be instrumental in scheduling family meetings and facilitating those meetings, and in helping parents understand how important it is for siblings to be involved as well. Just at a time when families with children recently diagnosed with special healthcare needs really need to keep their boundaries open to access the community resources that they need, some families close those boundaries due to grief, depression, or other emotions associated with this unexpected transition in their family journey.

Family ecological theory

This theory, sometimes called bioecological systems theory, had its orgins in the work of Urie Bronfenbrenner (in Addison, 1992), and has been revised to be useful in describing the complex layers of family environments that affect all members of the family system. The interaction between factors in the child's maturing biology, the child's immediate family/community environment, and the societal landscape fuels and steers the child's development. Changes in any layer, such as biology (the child or adolescent's diagnosis), the family or environment, or society will ripple throughout other layers. So, we must understand all of these potential changes to best target our care for the family as client.

Terminology

The *microsystem* – this layer includes relationships and interactions that a child has with the immediate family (Berk, 2000). Structures in the microsystem include family, school, neighborhood, or childcare environments. Relationships can be bidirectional: actions of family members affect a child but actions of the child can also affect the family. For example, a child with autism may not show the attachment cues to his or her parents, such as early social smiles, which can negatively affect parental bonding.

The *mesosystem* – this layer provides the connection between the structures of the child's microsystem (Berk, 2000). These connections, such as between family and school, family and religious institution, etc. need to be carefully assessed because it is often the strength or challenges in these relationships that predict how the family does.

The *exosystem* – this layer defines the larger social system in which the child does not function directly. The structures in this layer impact the child's development by interacting with some structure in his or her microsystem (Berk, 2000). Parent workplace schedules or community-based family resources are examples. Although the child or adolescent may not be directly involved at this level, the strengths and challenges that the family feels from this layer indirectly affect the child.

The *macrosystem* – this layer may be considered the outermost layer in the child's environment. Although not being a specific framework, this layer is comprised of cultural values, customs, and laws (Berk, 2000). The effects of larger principles defined by the macrosystem have a cascading influence throughout the interactions of all other layers. For example, fathers raising their children with special healthcare needs may not receive the same services as mothers might if the cultural belief is that this is the mother's job.

The *chronosystem* – this system encompasses the dimension of time as it relates to a child's environments. Elements within this system can be either external, such as the timing of a parent's death, or internal, such as the physiological changes that occur with the aging of a child. As children get older, their thinking and abilities are expected to become more complex, and they begin to be able to make decisions about how changes in their various subsystems will affect them. This expectable maturing, however, can be delayed or nonexistent when the child has severe intellectual disabilities, and this stagnation can put pressure on families and organizations that interact with children and adolescents.

Remember Mia, the 5–year-old with Down Syndrome whom we met in the introductory chapter? An optimal encounter with the healthcare system would have placed Mia in the center of multiple systems that directly and indirectly affected her well-being and that of her family, and might have eliminated an expensive, and potentially unnecessary, follow-up visit.

RESOURCES

Family assessment guidelines

- Family Social Network

  Family tradition

  Developmental stages

Household constellation/living environment

Space/privacy

Physical safety/comfort/accessibility

- Neighborhood environment

Stability and direction of change

Degree of homogeneity

Proximity and access to essential services

- Family Health

Strengths and challenges

Satisfaction with health behaviors

- Social and Financial Resources

Social support – open versus closed system

Availability and choices regarding leisure time

Adequacy of income sources for economic stability

Management of financial, legal, and protective affairs

- Life Style

Values/goals

Communication/decision making

Role/flexibility

(Based on work by Lapp et al., 1993, in Whyte (ed.), 1997, p. 12)

Family genograms and ecomaps

The genogram is very helpful in outlining the family's various internal and external structures (Wright & Leahy, 2005). Although one can use a computer program (such as this free genogram software found at http://www.progenygenetics.com/online-pedigree/), all one really needs to draw this picture of the family is a piece of paper and a pen. The genogram is a picture of the relationships among family members, and can convey a great deal of information in pictorial form. It is basically a family tree, and follows conventional symbolism. It is especially useful in a first contact with the family. In my practice of assessing children and adolescents who may have experienced abuse, doing a quick genogram helps me understand what family members the child may be talking about during disclosures. The genogram generally consists of two to three generations, and most families are eager to collaborate in developing this picture of their families. Here is an example of the standard symbols that are often used for genograms, including symbols for use with diverse families, families experiencing abuse, etc.

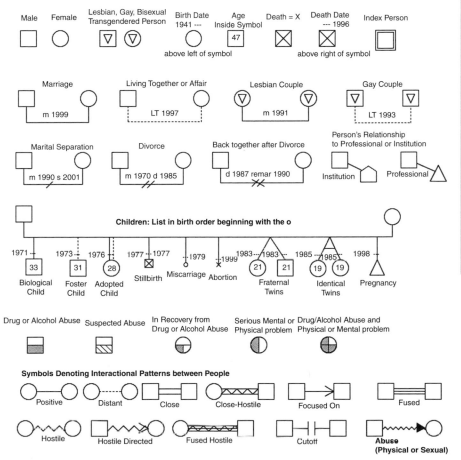

Figure 8.1 Standard Symbols for Genograms. Courtesy of Dr. Thomas Treadwell.

Identification of Family Composition

Family Member	Relationship in Family	Age Sex	Education	Occupation	Ethnicity	Social/Cultural Connections	Birth & development hx

Family Assessment Questions

	Findings
What are a couple of your goals for your family?	
How do you describe your family's culture?	
How will you help your foster child adapt to your culture?	
What does family mean to you?	
What are your hopes for your foster family?	
What are your biggest concerns in your family?	
When you have questions about parenting or need support, who can you turn to?	
How do you plan to provide for the basic needs for food, shelter, safety, and clothing for your foster child?	
How will you help your foster child adapt to the new environment that you are providing?	
How do you plan to honor potential spiritual or religious differences between you and your foster child?	
All families experience difficulties. Can you tell me about a difficulty that your family has faced and how it impacted the family?	

146

Family Assessment Questions	Findings
What characteristics would describe your family environment? How are the relationships among your family members/	
How accepting and supportive is your family toward foster care? What problems are you experiencing with the foster care system?	
How do you feel about the degree of attachment between you and your foster child?	
What ONE thing would you change about your current family situation if you had the opportunity? Why?	
I. Family Observations	
Does the family have financial resources to meet the needs of the family?	
What experience does the family have with being members of a foster family?	
What is the family health history? Are their unmet health care needs? Does chronic health or mental concerns, abuse (child abuse, sexual, domestic) substance abuse or special needs exist?	
In the family an open, closed or random social system? If open what are the external contacts and interactions?	
How has the family responded in the past to change?	
What are the cultural practices, beliefs, roles, view of children and parenting system?	
Summary of salient family goals.	

Summary of Current Family Functioning	Findings
What are the major areas of family concern at this time?	
What is the family's level of concern about these aspects of family life?	
How are these concerns impacting family processes?	
How successful is the family adapting to these impacts?	
How well is the family relating to external sources?	
Other	

Figure 8.2 (continued)

147

REFERENCES

Addison, J.T. (1992). Urie Bronfenbrenner. *Human Ecology, 20*(2), 16–20.

Berk, L.E. (2000). *Child development* (5th ed.) (pp. 23–38). Boston, MA: Allyn & Bacon.

Betz, C.L. (2000). California healthy and ready to work transition healthcare guide: Developmental guidelines for teaching health care self-care skills to children. *Issues in Comprehensive Pediatric Nursing, 23*, 203–244.

Erikson, E.H. (1963). *Childhood and society* (2nd ed.) New York, NY: WW Norton.

Lapp, C.A., Diemert, C.A., & Enestvedt, R. (1993). Family-based practice: Discussion of a tool merging assessment with intervention. In G.D. Wegner & R.J. Alexander (Eds.), *Readings in family nursing* (p. 100). Philadelphia, PA: Lippincott.

Pontious, S.L. (1982). Practical Piaget: Helping children understand. *American Journal of Nursing, 82*(1), 114–117.

Richmond, P.G. (1971). *An Introduction to Piaget.* New York, NY: Basic Books.

Rothman, J.G. (1989). Understanding of conservation of substance in youngsters with cerebral palsy. *Physical & Occupational Therapy in Pediatrics 9*(3), 119–125.

Whitchurch, G.G., & Constantine, L.L. (1993). Systems theory. In P.G. Boss, W.J. Doherty, R. LaRossa, et al. (Eds.), *Sourcebook of family theories and methods.* New York: Plenum Press.

Whyte, D.A. (1997). Explorations in family nursing. New York, NY: Routledge.

Wright, L.M., & Leahey, M. (2005). Nurses and families: A guide to family assessment and intervention. Philadelphia, PA: F.A. Davis.

USE OF THEORIES TO
GUIDE PRACTICE

CHAPTER 9

ENHANCING QUALITY OF LIFE FOR CHILDREN WITH SPECIAL HEALTHCARE NEEDS

Linda L. Eddy

This chapter incorporates current research to identify issues of health-related quality of life in children with disabilities and to offer suggestions to overcome some of the negative impact of chronic health problems on children and adolescents. Section headings include: (a) Quality of Life Defined, (b) Decreasing Pain, (c) Decreasing Fatigue, and (d) Resources.

QUALITY OF LIFE DEFINED

Quality of life (QOL) researchers have largely abandoned the notion that QOL and health-related quality of life are the same (Burckhardt & Anderson, 2003; Leplege & Hunt, 1997). Valid and reliable tools measuring general QOL have been in use since at least 1989 (see, e.g., Burckhardt, Woods, Schultz, & Ziebarth, 1989). There has been less attention paid to QOL in children, particularly children with chronic health problems, and definitional and measurement issues have yet to be resolved. The most comprehensive study of measures of the QOL of children who have chronic health problems occurred in the UK (Eiser & Morse, 2001). The authors systematically reviewed instruments designed to measure QOL and made recommendations regarding new measures of development and clinical applications. As part of this process, a number of formal approaches to the definition of QOL and its measurement were delineated. The sociological approach emphasizes the social and environmental aspects of QOL and the subjective nature of individual experience. The psychological approach emphasizes the role of individual appraisal in QOL. The medical approach, which draws on the above traditions, refers specifically to the impact of health and illness on the individual's QOL.

Scientific advances of the 20th century have resulted in more children with long-term physical and/or developmental problems surviving for longer periods of time, highlighting the need to consider quality as well as quantity of life. Significant definitional and measurement issues limit our understanding of children's QOL. One of the most serious is the tendency to use parent or clinician reports as patient proxies and the resulting and unsurprising disparity between adult and child perceptions of child QOL (Eiser & Morse, 2001).

Another issue is the use of disease-specific versus generic measures. Although disease-specific measures have the advantage of greater content validity, sensitivity, and specificity (Guyatt et al., 1989), generic measures allow for examination of QOL among children and adolescents with different conditions and allow for comparison to healthy populations. Most of the published research on childhood QOL assessed children with cancer or chronic illnesses, such as asthma and diabetes. There is little written about QOL in children with physical or developmental disabilities. We will examine both pain and fatigue as examples of symptoms that are related to decreased quality of life generally, and how they relate to children with special healthcare needs specifically.

DECREASING PAIN

Pain may be acute or chronic; it is perceived in response to acute tissue damage or even without actual stimulation. Undertreatment of pain is a serious worldwide public health crisis problem in the pediatric setting (Alexander & Manno, 2003). Poorly treated childhood pain can increase pain problems in adulthood, and we need to debunk old myths about pain in neonates and children that led to undertreatment (American Academy of Pediatrics/American Pain Society, 2001).

Pain assessment

Pain needs to be assessed and reassessed routinely, and pain assessment is multifactorial. There must be a focus on developmental influences on pain perception, physical indicators of pain, and, probably most important, a good understanding of the behavioral indicators of pain in children: restlessness, difficult to distract, irritability, grimacing, biting, posturing, drawing up knees, anorexia, lethargy, and sleep disturbances among many others. A pain history (from parent or other informant) is critical, especially in younger children or children with developmental or communication issues. This history should, at a minimum, include: typical expression of pain by this child, usual words used by this child for pain, previous experiences of pain and associated usual coping strategies, and preferences for analgesic treatment. It is unlikely that caregivers will be compliant with treatments with which they are uncomfortable, and often their discomfort can be at least partly ameliorated by good education.

As long as we are sensitive to developmental and communication needs for children, child self-reports of pain, fatigue, and other symptoms can be very helpful in a comprehensive pain assessment. The literature about the effectiveness of patient reported outcomes in children is complex. Current measurement of Patient Reported Outcomes (PROs) in children are limited. A variety of scales and other instruments are used in pain assessment for children, but most are lengthy & complex, and are adapted for use from adult measures (Canty-Mitchell, 2000). As part of a broad study on PROs in children with physical disabilities, Eddy and colleagues (2011) wanted to see how well youths were actually understanding the questions they were answering. After administering scales for children and adolescents to self-report their pain and fatigue, we asked them in follow-up cognitive interviews to tell us what they understood about the questions being asked on the scales. After the first 32 cognitive interviews, we noticed that many kids did not recognize terms, or misunderstood terms in scales. For example, when children and adolescents aged 8–20 were asked what they thought we meant by the word "average" when asked about their "average" level of pain, these study participants' answered varied widely. Examples included: "What most people are like" (12 yrs.), "Not at all" (10 yrs.), "Like, average is a lot and below average isn't", "Really painful" (9 yrs.), "Average means the total amount" (10 yrs.), and "You did OK" (20 yrs.). This demonstrates the need to be very clear when we are assessing symptoms in all children, and even more clear and sensitive to special needs children with this population. Overall, our study found that adult items and scales performed poorly in this population, and that younger participants (8–13 years) were twice as likely to answer "I don't know" to questions of word and construct meaning than older participants (14–20 years), who were more likely to guess.

It is also important to understand developmental level when asking for response options on assessment scales. In our study, (Eddy et al., 2011), both younger and older children were more accurate in their description of extremes such as "worst" and "least" than more ambiguous terms such as "average," and older participants had just as much difficulty making distinctions between response options such as "intense" and "severe" as did the younger group. Even with children who are able to understand how to respond to assessment questions, many answer particular questions even when they do not understand the question being asked. Because poorly constructed outcome measures hinder evaluation of nursing and other healthcare interventions, in developing simple, easily understood self-report measures there needs to be more of a focus on listening to the voices of children and youths with special needs.

In many clinical situations, use of a structured scale or instrument for pain assessment is not necessary, or its use can be supplemented by some broad, open-ended questions. Pain interview questions for children can include items such as: "Tell me about the hurt you are having now", or questions such as "How can I help you feel better right now?"

It is also important to consider cultural factors in pain assessment and management. Culture influences how pain is expressed, how much complaining is okay, and who is responsible for pain relief. Use words that have cross-cultural meaning, and when you do not know, ask! The resources section at the end of this chapter offers ideas and examples of appropriate pain assessment tools.

Pain management in children with special needs

The watchword in pain management is prevention, which depends heavily on the appropriate assessment discussed above. Pain relief, whether pharmacologic or non-pharmacologic, should be provided around-the-clock during periods of expected pain, and necessary medications should be administered orally or by IV if possible (Agency for Healthcare Policy and Research, 1992). Opioids are the mainstay for severe pain in children just as they are in adults, but pediatric healthcare providers are often hesitant to offer these medications. Just as with adults, the provider needs to observe for respiratory depression, especially during sleep, but this complication is most likely during initial administration of an opioid, and is no more likely to occur in a child than in an adult. The opioid of choice is often morphine, because meperidine's metabolites are known to be a source of seizures in some children, and may present an even greater threat in children with special healthcare needs that may predispose them to seizure development.

Mild-to-moderate pain and particularly pain related to inflammatory conditions will often respond well to the use of nonsteroidal anti-inflammatory medications, such as acetaminophen or ibuprofen. Although aspirin is given infrequently in childhood because of concerns about development of Reye's syndrome, children with juvenile rheumatoid arthritis (JRA) often respond well to aspirin, so education about avoiding aspirin use during times of viral illness must be included in patient education for children with JRA.

Within the context of a good assessment of need, desire, and development, non-pharmacologic pain management strategies are often quite effective with children, alone or as adjunct therapy (Agency for Healthcare Policy and Research, 1992). Examples included distraction; cutaneous stimulation (such as swaddle wrapping a young infant); relaxation strategies; and appropriate, cautious use of heat and cold applications. For example, a Finnish study (Axelin, Salanterä, Kirjavainen, & Lehtonen, 2009) compared FTP (facilitated tucking by parents), oral glucose administration, oral water administration as a placebo, and use of narcotics during painful procedures on preterm neonates (28–32 weeks). The authors found that FTP was preferable to all other pain management strategies studied when both efficacy and safety were examined.

Pain assessment and management specific to children with special needs

There is an evolving literature about specific pain assessment and management in children with special needs. For example, Engel and colleagues (2006) found that pain in individuals with cerebral palsy is often misattributed to the disability itself, is under-recognized and undertreated. These authors noted that the etiology of pain in individuals with cerebral palsy is multifactorial. Factors include hyperactive deep tendon reflexes and muscle spasm from spasticity, mobility limitations and resulting contractures, chronic overuse of available muscles and joints, and specific musculoskeletal deformities such as hip dysplasia. Most pain in children with cerebral palsy is chronic, and it occurs most often in the hip, knee, or foot, and is often reported in multiple sites. Challenges of pain assessment in this population include potential cognitive, motor, and communication impairments, difficulty differentiating involuntary muscle movements from pain grimacing, and lack of provider experience in caring for this population.

There are no published studies to date about effective pain management strategies targeted to the child or adolescent with cerebral palsy. The adult literature shows that many adults with cerebral palsy use passive strategies such as medication more often than active strategies such as biofeedback and cognitive behavioral therapy (Engel, Kartin, & Jensen, 2002), although the reason for this choice is not well understood. Medications considered potentially useful in the population range from narcotic analgesics to medications directed toward spasticity management such as botulinum toxin.

DECREASING FATIGUE

Attempts to isolate contributing factors to QOL in children with chronic health problems, particularly those with physical disabilities, generally center on pain (e.g., Engel, Petrina, Dudgeon, & McKearnan, 2005). Fatigue and its impact on general and health-related QOL in children is often forgotten or ignored. In fact, fatigue is a concept that has not been well studied in children at all (Farmer & Fowler, 2004). Our discussion of fatigue is heavily informed by work done by the author-editor and her colleagues in a systematic review of fatigue and its impact on quality of life in children with special healthcare needs (Eddy & Cruz, 2007).

There is no shared understanding of the meaning of fatigue to children. Some assessments query about general tiredness (Nagane, 2004; Petersen, Bergstrom, & Brulin, 2003). Others assess a child's level of energy for the completion of activities of daily living (Wilson, Yu, Goodnough, & Nissenson, 2004). The conceptualization of fatigue, especially with respect to measurement, is in its infancy. Many studies of children with chronic health problems do not ask about fatigue at all. When fatigue is considered, it is generally assessed as a dichotomous "yes–no" variable or measured on a visual analogue scale (Sallfors, Hallberg, & Fasth, 2004). One tool, the PedsQL Multidimensional Fatigue Scale, has been used across a few recent studies (Meeske et al., 2004; Varni, Burwinkle, & Szer, 2004), but is often completed by parents or clinicians as proxies. The extant literature documents significant discrepancies among parent, child, and clinician descriptions of fatigue (Hinds et al., 2000).

In addition, except for the research on cancer-related fatigue in children by Hinds et al. (2000) and Hinds and Hockenberry-Eaton (2001), most of the work in this area is outside of nursing and outside of the United States. Like QOL, most research that does take fatigue into account examines children with cancer (or, in some cases, with chronic fatigue syndrome), and there is little written about the fatigue as it impacts the QOL of children with physical or developmental disabilities.

The relative dearth of evidence related to fatigue in children with chronic health problems points to a gap in attention to this symptom. However, the pattern of fatigue as central to QOL in existing studies demonstrates that we need to elevate fatigue assessment and management to the level that we have achieved with pain. Hopefully, lessons learned in integrating pain assessment and management into the daily care of our young patients will inform our growing understanding of fatigue. Nurses and other healthcare providers have a perfect opportunity to notice situations resulting in fatigue and to document what works to alleviate that fatigue. In addition, we are attuned to listening to the stories of our young patients and to making clinical decisions based on those rich data. Paying attention to fatigue may go a long way toward alleviating it. For example, clustering interventions to allow for uninterrupted periods of rest or helping our young patients learn to plan their daily activities around their needs for balancing activity and rest will come more naturally as we begin to see fatigue reduction as central to increased QOL.

At this point, most of the evidence for specific fatigue-reducing interventions has been extrapolated from studies of fatigue in adults. However, some findings show promise for planning care of children and for further research related to childhood fatigue. For example, Kinsella (2002) found that behavioral interventions, including cognitive behavior therapy and graded exercise, had beneficial effects in reducing fatigue among people with chronic fatigue syndrome. These are interventions that can be modified, targeted toward children in both inpatient and outpatient settings, and tested for efficacy. The social isolation described by Johansson, Svensson, and Axelsson (2005) as a result of fatigue in patients with cancer needs to be considered in the lives of our child patients and routines adjusted to allow for desired social activities and contacts. The outcomes of a structured program to reduce fatigue in convalescing elderly adults showed that a combination of promoting nutrition, alternating periods of activity and rest, and offering gentle massage significantly reduced fatigue when compared to usual care (Robinson, Vollmer, & Hermes, 2003).

Programs for children with chronic health problems who are experiencing fatigue could include these interventions, and outcomes could be tested in this population. Finally, translation of evidence into changed practice necessitates teamwork. Children, families, and professionals need to reimagine ourselves as a team seeking to better understand how to improve the QOL of children with chronic health problems.

RESOURCES

Below is a link to an outstanding pain assessment and management module directed specifically toward the child or adolescent with special healthcare needs. The authors have given permission for this work to be copied and used freely. I have also included a link to the National Institutes of Health PROMIS (Patient Reported Outcomes Management Information Systems) web site where one can download scales to measure pain, fatigue, participation, and other facets of quality of life for children with a variety of special healthcare needs.

- **Pediatric Pain Assessment and Management Guide:** Developed by and available from the Oregon Center for Children and Youth with Special Health Needs located at the Child Development and Rehabilitation Center, Oregon Health & Science University, April 2011, in collaboration with nursing staff from OHSU, Multnomah County Health Department, Multnomah County Educational Service District, the Oregon Pain Commission, and a parent of two special needs children.

- **PROMIS Assessment Instruments Available for Download from the Assessment Center:** http://www.assessmentcenter.net/

REFERENCES

Agency for Healthcare Policy and Research, USDHHS.(1992). *Acute Pain Management Guideline Panel. Quick reference guide for clinicians number 1: Acute pain management in infants, children, and adolescents: Operative and medical Procedures.* Rockville, MD: US Dept of Health and Human Services, Agency for Health Care Policy and Research. AHCPR Publication No. 92-0020.

Alexander, J. & Manno, M. (2003). Underuse of analgesia in very young pediatric patients with isolated painful injuries. *Annals of Emergency Medicine, 41*(5), 617–622.

American Academy of Pediatrics (Committee on Psychosocial Aspects of Child and Family Health), American Pain Society (Task Force on Pain in Infants, Children, and Adolescents). (2001). The assessment and management of acute pain in infants, children, and adolescents. *Pediatrics*, 2001, 793–797.

Axelin, A., Salanterä, S., Kirjavainen, J., & Lehtonen, L. (2009). Oral glucose and parental holding preferable to opioid in pain management in preterm infants. *Clinical Journal of Pain, 25,* 138–145.

Burckhardt, C.S., & Anderson, K.L. (2003). The quality of life scale: Reliability, validity, and utilization. *Health Quality of Life Outcomes*, 1(1), 60.

Burckhardt, C.S., Woods, S.L., Schultz, A.A., & Ziebarth, D.M. (1989). Quality of life of adults with chronic illness: A psychometric study. *Research in Nursing & Health*, 12(6), 347–354.

Canty-Mitchell, J., & Zimet, G.D. (2000). Psychometric properties of the Multidimensional Scale of Perceived Social Support in urban adolescents. *American Journal of Community Psychology*, 28, 391–400.

Eddy, L.L., & Cruz, M. (2007). The relationship between fatigue and quality of life in children with chronic health problems: A systematic review. *Journal for Specialists in Pediatric Nursing*, 12(2), 105–114.

Eddy, L., Khastou, L., Cook, K., & Amtmann, D. (2011). Item selection in self-report measures for children and adolescents with disabilities: Lessons from cognitive interviews. *Journal of Pediatric Nursing*, 26, 559–565.

Eiser, C., & Morse, R. (2001). Quality of life measures in chronic diseases of childhood. *Health Technology Assessment,*5(4), 1–162.

Engel, J.M., Kartin, D., & Jensen, M.P. (2002). Pain treatment in persons with cerebral palsy: Frequency and helpfulness. *American Journal of Physical Medicine and Rehabilitation*, 81(4), 291–96. [PMID: 11953547] DOI:10.1097/00002060-200204000-00009.

Engel, J.M., Petrina, T.J., Dudgeon, B.J., & McKearnan, K.A. (2005). Cerebral palsy and chronic pain: A descriptive study of children and adolescents. *Physical & Occupational Therapy in Pediatrics*, 25(4), 73–84.

Engel, J.M., Jensen, M.P., & Schwartz, L. (2006). Coping with chronic pain associated with cerebral palsy. *Occupational Therapy International*, 13, 224–233.

Farmer, A., & Fowler, T. (2004). Prevalence of chronic disabling fatigue in children and adolescents. *British Journal of Psychiatry*, 18(4), 477–481.

Guyatt, G.H., Deyo, R.A., Charlson, M., et al. (1989). Responsiveness and validity in health-status measurement: A clarification. *Journal of Clinical Epidemiology*, 42(5), 254–268.

Hinds, P.S., & Hockenberry-Eaton, M. (2001). Developing a research program on fatigue in children and adolescents diagnosed with cancer. *Journal of Pediatric Oncology Nursing*, 18(2) Supplement 1, 3–12.

Hinds, P.S., Hockenberry-Eaton, M., Gilger, E., et al. (2000). Comparing patient, parent, and staff descriptions of fatigue in pediatric patients. *Cancer Nursing*, 22(4), 277–288.

Johansson, A., Svensson, E., & Axelsson, L. (2005). Social isolation: A nursing problem in cancer patients with fatigue. *Nursing Science & Research in the Nordic Countries*, 25(4), 60–63.

Kinsella, P. (2002). Review: Behavioural interventions show the most promise for chronic fatigue syndrome. *Evidence-Based Nursing*, 5(2), 46.

Leplege, A., & Hunt, S. (1997). The problem of quality of life in medicine. *Journal of the American Medical Association*, 278(1), 47–50.

Meeske, K., Katz, E.R., Palmer, S.N., et al. (2004). Parent proxy-reported health-related quality of life and fatigue in pediatric patients diagnosed with brain tumors and acute lymphoblastic leukemia. *Cancer*, 101(9), 2116–2125.

Nagane, M. (2004). Relationship of subjective chronic fatigue to academic performance. *Psychological Reports*, 95(1), 48–52.

Petersen, S., Bergstrom, E., & Brulin, C. (2003). High prevalence of tiredness and pain in young school children. *Scandinavian Journal of Public Health*, *31*, 367–374.

Robinson, S., Vollmer, C., & Hermes, B. (2003). A program to reduce fatigue in convalescing elderly adults. *Journal of Gerontological Nursing*, *29*(5), 47–53.

Sallfors, C., Hallberg, L.R., & Fasth, A. (2004). Well-being in children with juvenile chronic arthritis. *Clinical Expertise in Rheumatology*, *22*(1), 125–130.

Varni, J.W., Burwinkle, T.M., & Szer, I.S. (2004). The PedsQL Multideminsional Fatigue Scale in pediatric rheumatology: Reliability and validity. *Journal of Rheumatology*, *31*, 2494–2500.

Wilson, A., Yu, H.T., Goodnough, L.T., & Nissenson, A.R. (2004). Prevalence and outcomes of anemia in rheumatoid arthritis: A systematic review of the literature. *American Journal of Medicine*, *116* (Supplement 7A), 50S–57S.

ENHANCING QUALITY OF LIFE FOR CHILDREN WITH SPECIAL HEALTHCARE NEEDS

CHAPTER 10

IMPACT ON FAMILY AND INCREASING FAMILY WELL-BEING

Linda L. Eddy

Out of their own discomfort, healthcare providers often ignore or minimize needs of families of children with disabilities. I remember early in my career as a pediatric nurse practitioner sitting in the living room of a family with a 5-year-old child who was obviously delayed. I asked the family what it was like learning that their child had mental retardation. Immediately Derrick's mother said, "Mental retardation: now THAT is a word I can understand. His doctors just told us he had watershed injury to the brain or some such thing. Why can't you medical people use words we can understand?" It seemed inconceivable to me then that the family had lived with an unclear understanding of their child's special needs for five years. After thirty years in practice, though, I have seen this happen too many times.

This chapter will outline the critical nature of families and other caregivers in fostering the best possible outcomes for children and adolescents with special needs and for their families. We offer suggestions for enhancing family quality of life based on current research and clinical experience. Section headings are: (a) Family Well-Being, (b) Subjective Well-Being in Parents of Children with Disabilities; (c)Linking Family Well-Being to Child Well-Being, (d) Family Diversity and Well-Being, and (e) Making a Difference: Family Interventions. This chapter focuses on families of children with a broad range of chronic conditions that require care in excess of the demands of normal parenting (Stein & Jessop, 1982). We know that there are far more similarities than differences in family responses based on type of illness or disability (Konstantareas, Homitidis, & Plowright, 1992) but caring for children with behavior issues associated with chronic health problems increases parental burden and distress.

FAMILY WELL-BEING

The Healthy People 2010 national goal, to improve the health of children and adults with disabilities and to prevent secondary conditions (U.S. Department of Health & Human Services, 2006), has an objective that would have all 50 states and the District of Columbia providing public health surveillance and health promotion programs for persons with disabilities and their caregivers. This objective highlights the growing recognition of the importance of parental well-being in the lives of children with disabilities. In 2010, data from the national *Survey of Children with Special Health Care Needs* (HRSA, 20010) indicated that approximately 15% of children in the United States had special healthcare needs. With a population this large, clinicians might influence overall health with interventions that positively influence the well-being, levels of support, and stress levels of both children with disabilities and their parents. Taking a family approach is important both for the well-being of the child and his or her parents.

For the purposes of this chapter, we chose subjective well-being (SWB) to be one of the primary outcomes among parental caregivers. This emphasis is based on the ability of SWB and life satisfaction measures to predict long-term child and family functioning. SWB is also considered to be an important aspect of health-related quality of life (Camfield & Skevington, 2008), and in turn, health is an important determinant of subjective well-being (Helliwell & Putnam, 2004). Finally, a closely related concept to SWB, life satisfaction, has been shown to be related to health behaviors and health-related quality of life (Strine et al., 2008).

SWB can be reliably measured using brief self-report scales, such as the Satisfaction With Life Scale (SWLS) (Diener, Suh, & Oshi, 1997) suitable for use with children as well as adults. Brief, reliable and valid measures of quality of life have been developed and thus can be easily incorporated into a busy clinical practice (Zimmerman et al., 2006).

SUBJECTIVE WELL-BEING IN PARENTS OF CHILDREN WITH DISABILITIES

SWB refers quite generally to how people evaluate their lives (Diener, Suh, & Oishi, 1997) and taps relatively enduring self-reported feelings of well-being. Examples of items developed to measure SWB include: (a) in most ways my life is close to my ideal, (b) the conditions of my life are excellent, and (c) I am satisfied with my life (Pavot & Diener, 1993).

In *Children with Disabilities: A Longitudinal Study of Child Development and Parent Well-Being*, Hauser-Cram and colleagues (2001) examined the bidirectional relationship between parent well-being and child outcomes that affect school and life skills in children with Down syndrome, mobility impairment, and developmental delay of unknown etiology. They found that parent well-being and level of functioning predicted both mental age and adaptive behavior, and in turn children's mental age and behavior influenced parent well-being (Hauser-Cram, Warfield, Shokoff, & Krauss, 2001).

Numerous studies have documented the impact of children with chronic illnesses and disabilities on both individual parental outcomes, such as depression or life satisfaction, and dyadic outcomes, such as marital satisfaction or marital stability (e.g., Wallander & Varni, 1998). Few studies, however, have examined SWB as the construct of interest. When SWB has been studied, positive as well as negative perceptions of well-being have been documented. For example, King, Scollon, Ramsey, & Williams (2000) found that parents of children with Down syndrome were more likely to describe high levels of SWB if their stories included foreshadowing of the event and self-described happy endings. In a

IMPACT ON FAMILY AND
INCREASING FAMILY WELL-BEING

study of SWB and other variables in parents of children with developmental disabilities, higher levels of positive reappraisal of the situation were associated with higher levels of SWB, whereas higher levels of escape or avoidance were associated with lower levels of maternal SWB (Glidden, Billings, & Jobe, 2006). Similarly, Dudevany and Abboud (2003) found that the higher the amount of informal support resources, the higher the sense of maternal well-being.

Studies examining the effects of parenting children with disabilities on outcomes related to SWB, such as relationship quality, report mixed findings. An early critique concluded that parents of children with chronic illnesses experienced more marital distress than other parents (Sabbeth & Leventhal, 1984). However, a later review found evidence of both positive and negative effects on the marital dyad (Benson & Gross, 1989). Several studies (e.g., Abbott & Meredith, 1986; Kazak, 1987), however, found no differences in marital satisfaction between parents caring for children with chronic health problems and those caring for well children. Because these studies involved small clinical samples, Eddy and Walker (1999) examined marital satisfaction and stability using a large, nationally representative sample. Significantly, they found no differences on either measure between parents caring for children with chronic health problems and those with well children.

Nonmarital effects on the family unit have been studied less widely. Although a few studies have documented family concerns about social isolation and other psychosocial outcomes (e.g., Abresch, Seyden, & Wineinger, 1998; Bothwell et al., 2002; Jenney & Campbell, 1997), at least one study found no differences between families of children with chronic health problems and families of well children on a variety of family-functioning measures. Magill-Evans et al. (2001) found that families of adolescents and young adults with cerebral palsy demonstrated similar scores on family functioning and life satisfaction as families of adolescents without a disability

There is evidence that in certain cases the type and severity of disability is related to parental functioning. For example, in a study of the health and well-being of caregivers of children with cerebral palsy, behavioral problems and the level of caregiver burden had negative direct effects on family functioning, and indirect negative effects on caregiver psychological and physical health (Raina et al., 2005). Similarly, behavioral issues in children with developmental disabilities seemed to be clear and consistent predictors of high stress levels in caregivers (Friedrich, Cohen, & Wilturner, 1987; Singer & Farkas, 1989; Woolfson, 2004). Some researchers such as Pless and Pinkerton (1975), however, suggest that illness chronicity has a greater impact on the child, parents, and siblings than the specific character of the disorder. Also, findings from a longitudinal study of the impact of type of illness or disability on children and their families differentiated families with children with chronic health problems from families of well children, but did not differentiate families of chronically ill children from families of developmentally disabled children (Stein & Jessop, 1982). More recently, Wallander and Varni (1998) found that neither the nature of the child's impairment (whether motor, speech, hearing or cognitive), nor its severity was associated with maternal adjustment.

LINKING FAMILY WELL-BEING TO CHILD WELL-BEING

There is an increasing body of literature about subjective well-being in children and adolescents. We know, for instance, that the quality of relationships with adults and peers at school is a protective factor for subjective well-being in children, whereas depression and anxiety are risk factors for decreased levels of subjective well-being (Lindberg & Swanberg, 2006). A Finnish study found that self-perceived satisfaction with school, with body image, and with health predicted high levels of overall SWB in young adolescents. High levels of drinking, poor health, and lack of satisfaction with school predicted lower SWB (Rask, Astedt-Kurki, Paavilainen, & Laippala, 2003). In a study of familial contributions to adolescent SWB (Joronen & Astedt-Kurki, 2005), teens described feeling valued by their parents as contributing to well-being whereas excessive dependency on parents was one of the contributors to ill-being. These and other studies point to the need to enhance positive attitudes in children and adolescents, and to teach them strategies to cope with negative emotions and to live as independently as possible.

A considerable body of literature has documented the effects of childrearing on the SWB of parents in the general population. For example, Ishil-Kuntz and Ihinger-Tallman (1991) compared effects of marital and parental status on three domains of well-being, including global life satisfaction, and found that first-married biological parents reported greater satisfaction with parenting than did remarried biological parents and stepparents. The literature on transition to parenthood consistently documents an array of negative individual and family outcomes occurring after the birth of a first child (Cowan & Cowan, 1995), whether that outcome is decline in marital quality (Demo & Cox, 2000), increased risk for psychological symptoms (Cox, Paley, Burchinal, & Payme, 1999), or disrupted support structures (Cowan & Cowan).

There is a growing understanding of the close ties between parent well-being and child well-being. A 2003 study (Rask et al.) of the relationship of family dynamics to SWB found that high levels of family stability and mutuality and low levels of family problems predicted high levels of global life satisfaction in a sample of 239 seventh and ninth grade students, whereas serious family problems, family disorganization, and family illness were highly related to subjective ill-being. Knoester (2003) assessed the extent to which changes in

IMPACT ON FAMILY AND
INCREASING FAMILY WELL-BEING

the psychological well-being of young adults engendered changes in their parents' psychological well-being, and vice versa. The results suggested that the relationship is reciprocal: changes in a young adult's psychological well-being affect the psychological well-being of a parent. Similarly, changes in a parent's feelings of well-being affect those of a young adult offspring. The National Survey of Child and Adolescent Well-Being examined parent and child outcomes in families who came into contact with the Child Welfare System and linked caregiver mental and physical health as well as services received to level of caregiver well-being and ability to provide the supportive relationships that children need for their development and well-being (US Department of Health & Human Services, 2005).

FAMILY DIVERSITY AND WELL-BEING

Often, a discussion of family diversity is more of a discussion of best practices in caring for families for whom English is a nonnative language. Although this discussion is very important, looking at culture and diversity more broadly can sensitize the nurse to a broad range of culture issues in families. The definition of culture suggested by the Nurturing Cultural Competence in Nursing program, funded by the Robert Wood Johnson Foundation and the Northwest Health Foundation's Partners Investing in Nursing's Future (PIN) program, and including research by the editor, will be used as the working definition of culture in this text. Cultural competence is thus defined as: *A lifelong process of examining values and beliefs and developing an inclusive approach to practice with active intercultural engagement.* This definition reflects a broad description of culture that includes, but is not limited to, age, gender, race, ethnicity, religion, sexual orientation, socioeconomic status, and physical or mental abilities.

Disparities related to race, ethnicity, and socioeconomic status are still prevalent in the American healthcare system. The Institute of Medicine's seminal publication, *Unequal Treatment* (2002) reports "the vast majority of published research indicates that minorities are less likely than whites to receive needed services, including clinically necessary procedures, even after correcting for access-related factors, such as insurance status." In addition to ethnic groups, other groups face health disparities based on gender, religion, and sexual orientation, among others.

Few studies examine the association between race and ethnicity and outcomes in families of children with disabilities (Eddy & Engel, 2008). However, in one study examining families with deaf children, ethnicity was not related to parents' stress level (Pipp-Siegel, Sedey, & Yoshinaga-Itano, 2002). The authors suggest that this finding in their sample may be a result of low overall stress and high support. The influence of income on families of children with disabilities has been studied more often than the influence of ethnicity (Eddy & Engel). Several studies found that gross income was positively related to family health, although there were general cost-related concerns and resulting stress in most families (Bothwell et al., 2002; Dobson & Middleton, 1998). In one study that examined effects of ethnicity and socioeconomic resources on the well-being of mothers of young adults with intellectual disabilities (Eisenhower & Blacher, 2006), higher well-being scores for Caucasian mothers compared to Latina mothers was entirely explained by socioeconomic status. Thus, family-level interventions for parents of children with disabilities have to consider resource costs and availability if they are to be useful for this population.

MAKING A DIFFERENCE: FAMILY INTERVENTIONS

Culturally sensitive interventions

The previous sections indicate that families who have children with disabilities are likely to experience threats to their well-being both individually and collectively. Such families could conceivably benefit from education and support interventions that provide forums for learning as well as for receiving support from healthcare providers and other families experiencing similar issues. Supportive interventions that work for families must be informed by cultural awareness, whether we are talking about race, ethnicity, socioeconomic status, gender, sexual orientation, or any other family variable. Easily available interventions aimed at caring for individuals and families across cultures can be found on the following web site: http://www.ocnnursingdiversity.org/documents/NCCNProgram2010.pdf.

As just one example, this project developed an online cultural competence tutorial focusing on two ethnic groups commonly encountered in the United States. Two cultural consultants with expertise in Latino and Native American cultures participated in the development of the tutorial. The tutorial consists of three one–hour modules. **Module One:** *Aspects of Cultural Assessment* focuses on discussion of general aspects of cultural beliefs and practices, which are incorporated into an assessment to determine their impact on health beliefs, decisions, and practices. **Module Two:** *Caring for the Hispanic Client* outlines changing ethic demographies and discusses cultural beliefs and practices of Hispanic Americans that may impact their health beliefs, decisions, and practices. Similarly, **Module Three:** *Caring for the Native American Client,* has as its objectives the describing of various Native American tribes and discussing cultural beliefs and practices of Native Americans that may impact their health beliefs, decisions, and practices.

Flexible interventions

Overall, it is clear that programs that work for families of children with disabilities need to be sensitive to differing family needs and flexible enough to accommodate change over time. In a recent article (Eddy & Engel, 2008), the editor and her colleague suggested a program that was flexible enough to offer services to families with children with a variety of disabilities and that could be initiated at any point in the healthcare system. (For more information, see original publication, Eddy & Engel, in *Rehabilitation Nursing*.)

The authors found that families of children with special healthcare needs required a care team that was able to recognize when care needs intensify. For this reason, child healthcare team members need to work together to assure that a comprehensive pediatric healthcare "home" is available to all families with youths with special needs. The healthcare home, according to the National Association of Pediatric Nurse Practitioners (2001), is a place where children and families receive, among other things, health promotion, advocacy for parenting, anticipatory guidance, consultation on developmental and behavioral issues, and assistance with connection to community resources.

Arguably, the healthcare home need not be as much a geographic "place" as a team of professionals dedicated to coordinated care for families of children with disabilities. Eddy and Engel (2008) proposed such a model: the family HOMETEAM. The HOMETEAM would include usual aspects of care coordination such as assessment, planning, implementation, evaluation, monitoring, support, education, and advocacy (Lindeke, Leonard, Presler, & Garwick, 2002) but would differ in that the single point of contact would be the HOMETEAM rather than a single healthcare professional. The team, a small group of professionals headed by the family and in regular communication, could interact flexibly to meet ongoing and changing needs. Team composition would be dependent on family needs, and might change over time.

Families who have ongoing worry about their child's physical or emotional well-being or who are unable to participate in normal family activities may feel isolated and lack knowledge about what kinds of resources are available or how to get connected with those resources. The HOMETEAM could facilitate access to services that help to increase the child's health and decrease family worry, activity limitation, and activity interruption. Stewardship of resources would be facilitated by plans individually geared for the family so that needs are met but resources are not wasted. This might take the form of increased access

IMPACT ON FAMILY AND INCREASING FAMILY WELL-BEING

to specialized healthcare providers and therapists for some families, whereas others would be best served by help with finding outlets for mobility aids, access to respite services, or connection with specialized daycare settings.

Needless to say, these are expensive services, and any comprehensive plan of care must include financial advocacy for families. The isolation and lack of access to care that are common in families with children with disabilities may be intensified for families with limited incomes. These are areas that might respond to sensitive, culturally competent, knowledgeable interventions from the HOMETEAM. Ensuring the sensitivity and appropriateness of care can be fostered by placing families at the center of the team, planning toward family strengths rather than deficits, and considering broader issues of policy development and attention to population health.

REFERENCES

Abbott, D.A., & Meredith, W.H. (1986). Strengths of parents with retarded children. *Family Relations: Journal of Applied Family & Care Studies, 35*(3), 371–375.

Abresch, R.T., Seyden, N.K., & Wineinger, M.A. (1998). Quality of life: Issues for persons with neuromuscular diseases. *Physical Medicine and Rehabilitation Clinics of North America, 1998*(9), 233–248.

Benson, B.A., & Gross, A.M. (1989). The effect of a congenitally handicapped child upon the marital dyad: A review of the literature. *Clinical Psychology Review, 9,* 747–758.

Bothwell, J.E., Dooley, J.M., Gordon, K.E., et al. (2002). Duchenne Muscular Dystrophy – parental perceptions. *Clinical Pediatrics, 41*(2), 105–109.

Camfield, L., & Skevington, S.M. (2008). On subjective well-being and quality of life. *Journal of Health Psychology, 13*(6), 764–775.

Child and Adolescent Health Measurement Initiative (CAHMI). (2009–2010). National Survey of Children with Special Health Care Needs Indicator Data Set. Data Resource Center for Child and Adolescent Health.

Cowan, C.P., & Cowan, P.A. (1995). Interventions to ease the transition to parenthood: Why they are needed and what they can do. *Family Relations, 44,* 412–423.

Cox, M.J., Paley, B., Burchinal, M., & Payne, C.C. (1999). Marital perceptions and interactions across the transition to parenthood. *Journal of Marriage and the Family, 61,* 611–625.

Demo, D.H., & Cox, M.J. (2000). Families with young children: A review of research in the 1990s. *Journal of Marriage and the Family, 62,* 876–895.

Diener, E., Suh, E.M., & Oishi, S. (1997). Recent findings on subjective well-being. *Indian Journal of Clinical Psychology, 24*(1), 25–41.

Dobson, B., & Middleton, S. (1998). *Paying to care: The cost of childhood disability.* York, UK: Joseph Rowntree Foundation.

Dudevany, I., & Abboud, S. (2003). Stress, social support and well-being of Arab mothers of children with intellectual disability who are served by welfare services in northern Israel. *Journal of Intellectual Disability Research, 47,* 264–272.

Eddy, L.L., & Walker, A.J. (1999). The impact of children with chronic health problems on marriage. *Journal of Family Nursing, 5*(1), 10–32.

Eddy, L.L., & Engel, J.M. (2008). The impact of child disability type on the family. *Rehabilitation Nursing, 33*(3), 98–103.

Eisenhower, A., & Blacher, J. (2006). Mothers of young adults with intellectual disability: Multiple roles, ethnicity and well-being. *Journal of Intellectual Disability Research, 50*(12), 905–916.

Friedrich, W.N., Cohen, D.S., & Wilturner, L.S. (1987). Family relations and marital quality when a mentally handicapped child is present. *Psychological Reports, 61*, 911–919.

Glidden, L.M., Billings, F.J., & Jobe, B.M. (2006). Personality, coping style and well-being of parents rearing children with developmental disabilities. *Journal of Intellectual Disability Research, 50*, 949–962.

Hauser-Cram, P., Warfield, M.E., Shokoff, J.P., & Krauss, M.W. (2001). Results: Predictors of functioning and change in children's development and parent well-being. In W.F. Overton (Ed.), Children with disabilities: A longitudinal study of child development and parent well-being. *Monographs of the Society for Research in Child Development, 54*–78.

Helliwell, J.F., & Putnam, R.D. (2004). The social context of well-being. *Philosophical Transitions. Royal Society of London, 359*, 1435–1445.

Institute of Medicine. (2002). Unequal treatment: Confronting racial and ethnic disparities in healthcare. B.D. Smedley, A.Y. Smith, & A.R. Nelson (Eds.). Washington, DC: National Academies Press.

Ishil-Kuntz, M., ∗ Ihinger-Tallman, M. (1991). The subjective well-being of parents. *Journal of Family Issues, 12*(1), 58–68.

Jenney, M.E., & Campbell, S. (1997). Measuring quality of life. *Archives of Disease in Childhood, 77*, 347–350.

Joronen, K., & Astedt-Kurki, P. (2005). Familial contribution to adolescent subjective well-being. *International Journal of Nursing Practice, 11*, 125–133.

Kazak, A.E. (1987). Families with disabled children: Stress and social networks in three samples. *Journal of Abnormal Child Psychology, 15*, 137–146.

King, L.A., Scollon, C.K., Ramsey, C., & Williams, T. (2000). Stories of life transition: Subjective well-being and ego development in parents of children with Down syndrome. *Journal of Research in Personality, 34*, 509–536.

Knoester, C. (2003). Transitions in young adulthood and the relationship between parent and offspring well-being. *Social Forces, 81*(4), 1431–1457.

Konstantareas, M.M., Homatidis, S., & Plowright, C.M. (1992). Assessing resources and stress in parents of severely dysfunctional children through the Clarke modification of Holroyd's Questionnaire on Resources and Stress. *Journal of Autism & Developmental Disorders, 22*(2), 217–234.

Lindberg, L., & Swanberg, I. (2006). Well-being of 12-year-old children related to interpersonal relations, health habits and mental distress. *Scandinavian Journal of Caring Sciences, 20*, 274–281.

Lindeke, L.L., Leonard, B.J., Presler, B., & Garwick, A. (2002). Family-centered care coordination for children with special needs across multiple settings. *Journal of Pediatric Health Care, 16*(6), 290–297.

Magill-Evans, J., Darrh, J., Pain, K., et al. (2001). Are families with adolescents and young adults with cerebral palsy the same as other families? *Developmental Medicine & Child Neurology, 43*, 466–472.

IMPACT ON FAMILY AND INCREASING FAMILY WELL-BEING

National Association of Pediatric Nurse Practitioners (2001). *Position statement on access to care*. Retrieved from http://www.napnap.org

Pavot, W., & Diener, E. (1993). Review of the Satisfaction With Life Scale. *Psychological Assessment, 5*, 164–172.

Pipp-Siegel, S., Sedey, A.L., & Yoshinaga-Itano, C. (2002). Predictors of parental stress in mothers of young children with hearing loss. *Journal of Deaf Studies and Deaf Education, 7*(1), 1–17.

Pless, I.B., & Pinkerton, P. (1975). *Chronic childhood disorder: Promoting patterns of adjustment*. London, UK: Jerry Kimpton.

Raina, P., O'Donnell, M., Rosenbaum, P., et al. (2005). The health and well-being of caregivers of children with cerebral palsy. *Pediatrics, 115*, 1755.

Rask, K., Astedt-Kurki, P., Paavilainen, E., & Laippala, P. (2003). Adolescent subjective well-being and family dynamics. *Scandinavian Journal of Caring Sciences, 17*, 129–138.

Sabbeth, B.F., & Leventhal, J.M. (1984). Marital adjustment to chronic childhood illness: A critique of the literature. *Pediatrics, 73*, 762–768.

Singer, L., & Farkas, K.J. (1989). The impact of infant disability on maternal perception of stress. *Family Relations, 38*, 444–449.

Stein, R.E., & Jessop, D. (1982). A noncategorical approach to chronic childhood illness. *Public Health Reports, 97*, 354–362.

Strine, T.W., Chapman, D.P., Balluz, L.S., et al. (2008). The associations between life satisfaction and health-related quality of life, chronic illness, and health behaviors among U.S. community-dwelling adults. *Journal of Community Health, 33*(1), 40–50.

US Department of Health & Human Services. (2005). National survey of child and adolescent well-being. Retrieved from http://www.acf.hhs.gov/programs/opre/abuse_neglect/nscaw/reports/cps_sample/cps_ch11.html

US Department of Health & Human Services. (2006). *Healthy people 2010 midcourse review*. Retrieved from http://www.healthypeople.gov/data/midcourse/default.htm#pubs

Wallander, J., & Varni, J. (1998). Effects of paediatric chronic physical disorders on child and family adjustment. *Journal of Child Psychology and Psychiatry, 39*, 29–46.

Woolfson, L. (2004). Family well-being and disabled children: A psychosocial model of disability-related child behaviour problems. *British Journal of Health Psychology, 9*,1–13.

Zimmerman, M., Ruggero, C.J., Chelminski, I., et al. (2006). Developing brief scales for use in clinical practice: The reliability and validity of single-item self-report measures of depression symptom severity, psychosocial impairment due to depression, and quality of life. *Journal of Clinical Psychiatry, 67*, 1536–1541.

IMPACT ON FAMILY AND
INCREASING FAMILY WELL-BEING

PUBLIC HEALTH AND SCHOOL HEALTH NURSING OF CHILDREN WITH SPECIAL HEALTHCARE NEEDS

Phyllis Eide

COMMUNITY HEALTH NURSING WITH CHILDREN WITH SPECIAL HEALTH NEEDS

Assuring adequate maternal child health (MCH) is a key factor in laying the foundation for healthy adulthood. Two areas of nursing practice of MCH, and the subset population of children with special health needs, are school health nursing and public health nursing. This chapter will review the historical context of both areas of nursing as they relate to care of children with special health needs, followed by a discussion of the varying roles associated with public health and school health. The federal Maternal and Child Health Bureau's definition of children with special needs is adopted for the purposes of this chapter: "children who have or are at increased risk for a chronic physical, developmental, behavioral or emotional condition, and who also require health care–related services of a types of amount beyond that required by children generally" (van Dyck et al., 2004). Another term found in the literature describing the children in this population is a reference to *medically fragile* children (Mentro, 2003). A discussion of case management and evidence-based home visiting programs will be included, along with a review of key resources available to professionals and families of children with special health needs.

PUBLIC HEALTH AND CHILDREN WITH SPECIAL HEALTH NEEDS

The pre-eminent federal legislation of the 20th century that had the greatest impact on maternal child health was the 1935 Social Security Act's Title V. However, the ground for this legislation was laid by two prior entities in the early years of the 20th century. In 1912, the Federal Children's Bureau was created to "investigate and report on the status of children and on their common as well as special needs" and on "the welfare of children and child life among all classes of our people" (About Title V, n.d.). This resulted in child labor laws, establishment of maternal health standards, the school lunch program, and uniform birth registration. The Sheppard-Towner Maternity and Infancy Act of 1921 carried the work forward by providing the first federal grants to states for public health. Opposition to this "socialistic" and "radical" act, led by such groups as the Catholic Church, the Public Health Service, and the American Medical Association (AMA), led to the act's repeal in 1929. The American Academy of Pediatrics was formed in 1930, born in protest of the AMA's role in the Act's repeal (About Title V).

The stage, now set with a new focus on child welfare and rights, was established by the Children's Health Bureau and the Sheppard-Towner Act (1921); however briefly, both forged the way for federal assistance to states on specific health issues and for distinct populations. In the depths of the

Depression, the 1935 Social Security Act contained eleven Titles, primarily covering aid to the elderly, the unemployed, dependent children, and maternal child health (Legislative History: 1935 Social Security Act, n.d.). Title V, Section 511 created Services for Crippled Children (later renamed Children with Special Health Care Needs), providing federal funding and requiring state financial participation. By 1938, only one state lacked a Crippled Children's program (Understanding Title V of the Social Security Act, n.d.).

In the 1950s, special federal funding was allocated for projects targeting the "mentally retarded" (known as "MR funds") (Understanding Title V of the Social Security Act, n.d.). In 1981, the Maternal Child block grant approach was adopted, with the Children with Special Health Needs (CSHN) identified as part of the direct care services category in the MCH Block grant (Title V: Maternal and Child Health Services Block Grant Program, n.d.). This program falls under the Maternal Child Health Bureau, which is a part of the Health Resources and Services Administration (HRSA) (Understanding Title V of the Social Security Act, n.d.).

One of the several overarching goals of Title V includes facilitating the development of comprehensive, family-centered, community-based, culturally competent, coordinated systems of healthcare for children with special health needs. The following section illustrates some of the resources and systems of care available to nurses and families with special health needs children.

PUBLIC HEALTH AND COMMUNITY HEALTH PROGRAMS SERVING THIS SPECIAL NEEDS POPULATION

A good place to start when looking for state or jurisdiction contacts for the CSHCN programs can be found at HRSA's Maternal Child Health Bureau web site (http://mchb.hrsa.gov/). This site has a search engine that will allow you to enter your state or jurisdiction's name, and yields contact information on the state or jurisdictional official associated with the CSHN program. At the state level, you can find official web sites dedicated to CHSN, such as this one for the State of Washington: http://www.doh.wa.gov/YouandYourFamily/InfantsChildrenandTeens/HealthandSafety/ChildrenwithSpecialHealthCareNeeds.aspx. Such sites can function as portals to a wide array of services and resources available to healthcare providers and families with children who have special health needs. Expanded information and resource directories localized to specific counties can be found at many county health department web sites. Here are some examples:

The Spokane Regional Health District (SRHD), in Spokane, WA has a web site that provides information on the Infant Toddler network, which is designed to give assistance to families with children from birth to age 3 who have developmental delays or have a condition that might result in a developmental delay. Children with vision and/or hearing loss may also be qualified for help. Family resource coordinators help families coordinate evaluations and assessments, and serve as a single point of contact for a variety of services and liaison to other healthcare providers. These coordinators also assist families in developing an Individualized Family Service Plan (IFSP) (http://www.srhd.org/services/itn.asp)

The Seattle/King County, Washington public health department's web site provides a link to public health centers located throughout the Seattle and King County area, and lists the identification of special needs for a child with disabilities or special health concerns, with subsequent provision of information, support, and referrals, as one of their listed services (www.kingcounty.gov/healthservices/health/locations/phn.aspx).

The Snohomish, Washington county health department site not only has a special page for children with special health care needs, but has also produced a family-friendly brochure outlining what the program is and who is eligible, and providing examples of types of conditions covered, an outline of what services are available, and a clear presentation of how referrals can be made (including contact information) (http://www.snohd.org)

Public health nurses involved with CSHCN programs routinely coordinate and connect with community-based or population-based resources. One example of this type of resource is the Easter Seals organization, which provides "exceptional services to ensure that people with disabilities and families in need have equal opportunities to live, learn, work and play" (http://wa.easterseals.com/). These services include help with assistive technology devices, and camping and respite programs with barrier-free environments for children and adults, allowing the experience of all aspects of camping without the usual limitations. Child development services and workforce development initiatives are also components of the Easter Seals programs. Camping information for Washington State is also available through the Center for Children with Special Needs, a resource available through the Seattle Children's Hospital (http://cshcn.org/) that was established in 1998 to serve the needs of children and families throughout the greater Pacific Northwest and Alaska.

Public health nurses who work in areas with a high concentration of military families may collaborate with on-base programs and initiatives such as the Defense Department's Exceptional Family Member program. With over 100,000 military families with a special needs member, concerns about rotations and deployments, particularly in regards to uprooting the CSHCN child from his or her current programs, can add stress and worry to the military

PUBLIC HEALTH AND SCHOOL
HEALTH NURSING

family. The Exceptional Member Program provides critical information about services, supports, and entitlements (Military Homefront, n.d.).

The Internet provides public health nurses and families access to exceptional sites such as the Family Village, sponsored by the Waisman Center of the University of Wisconsin/Madison (Family Village, n.d.). Billed as a "global community of disability-related resources," the site contains informational resources on such topics as specific diagnoses, communication connections, adaptive products and technology, adaptive recreational activities, education, worship, health issues, and disability-related media and literature.

Because of the overwhelming mass of information available on the Internet, public health nurses can assist CSHCN families to develop discernment in determining what sites have credible information and what sites may not be reliable. For example, sites whose URL address ends in ".gov" represents a governmental agency, and would be, generally speaking, more reliable than a site ending in ".com" – which denotes a commercial site. Site addresses ending in ".org" may also be more reliable, especially if connected to nationally recognized organizations and groups linked to the CSHCN population.

In the following section, the multitude of roles involved with public health and community health nursing of this CSHCN population will be explored, with linkage to nationally recognized standards of public health nursing care, and nationally established healthcare goals enshrined in the document *Healthy People 2010.*

COMMUNITY HEALTH NURSING ROLES WITH CHILDREN WITH SPECIAL HEALTH NEEDS

The framework used for the following discussion of community health nursing roles will utilize a nationally known model for public health practice: the Minnesota "wheel" model (Public Health Nursing Section, 2001). An additional resource is the *Public Health Nursing Standards: Scope and Standards of Practice*, published in 2007 by the American Nurses Association.

Children with special health needs (CSHCN) vary in the types and frequencies of services needed. Some may only need periodic screening and monitoring, and can be adequately managed via the medical or healthcare provider "home." Other children may require specialty or subspecialty care, treatments with complex medical devices, and a challenging regimen of medications. The CSHCN population is considered by some to be a vulnerable population that uses numerous healthcare services for overall wellness (Mentro, 2003).

Coordination of services for the child and family may require coordination with other community-based agencies and other medical providers, inclusion of early intervention services, and connection with school-based special education services (Center for Children with Special Needs, n.d.). Early intervention services may include assistive technology devices and services, vision and hearing services, social work services, speech/language therapy, family training/counseling and home visits, psychological services, and transportation services to address access issues (Spokane Regional Health District, n.d.).

Factors that may contribute to the vulnerability of the child with special needs and his/her family include poverty, social isolation secondary to additional caregiving demands imposed by the child's condition, and increased job mobility, which may dictate moving a significant distance from the usual family and friends' circle of support (Johnson, Kastner, & Committee/Section on Children with Disabilities, 2005, p. 507).

The Minnesota model's element of *collaboration* is an appropriate connection to these activities. Collaboration is defined as committing two or more persons or organizations to achieve a common goal through enhancing the capacity of one or more of them to promote and protect health (Public Health Nursing Section, 2001). This role is also specified as Standard #11 for public health nurses (American Nurses Association, 2007b), but with a focus of work at the population level. Such activities could include partnering with other disciplines to engage in the activities of assessing, planning, implementing, and evaluating population-focused policies, programs, and services (American Nurses Association, p. 32).

Because societal factors and individual circumstances may sometimes strain a family's ability to provide for their child's special needs (Johnson et al., 2005, p. 507), it is critical that necessary resources are enhanced by interprofessional/multidisciplinary collaboration and prevention of duplicative services. In the process of collaboration, the participants must be willing to be potentially transformed or changed themselves through their involvement with collective goals that exceed individual interests (Public Health Nursing Section, 2001).

The public health nursing role of *advocate* is also frequently brought to bear in working with families with special healthcare needs children. In the Minnesota model of public health nursing practice, *advocacy* is defined as the ability to "plead someone's cause, or act on someone's behalf, with a focus on developing the community, system, individual, or family's capacity to plead their own cause or act on their own behalf" (Public Health Nursing Section, 2001, p. 263).

Because of the many complex and confusing systems, bureaucracies, and services, families are vulnerable to the desire to abdicate decision making to the professionals. Public health nurses and other healthcare providers

PUBLIC HEALTH AND SCHOOL
HEALTH NURSING

involved with these families must gently resist this impulse on the part of the family, while steadily and carefully working to craft a partnership with the family that will empower them to make their own choices and decisions, with guidance and input as appropriate. The role of *advocate* should not supplant the family's own voice and role, but rather should provide the opportunity to tie advocacy to other interventions such as referral and follow-up, community organizing, and policy development and enforcement (Public Health Nursing Section, 2001, p. 264).

Advocacy comprises Public Health Nurses' Standard #16, and is defined as an action that is taken to protect the health, safety, and rights of the population (American Nurses' Association, 2007b). Advocates need to know, when taking risks, what the difference is between rule bending and rule breaking, and that seeking a win-win circumstance is the ideal whenever possible (Public Health Nursing Section, 2001, p. 266).

CASE MANAGEMENT WITH CHILDREN WITH SPECIAL HEALTH NEEDS

Collaborative action is taken on issues that matter to all involved. Within a context of *case management*, which is a process that optimizes the self-care abilities of individuals and families, community-based nurses and other healthcare providers can collaborate on service delivery to prevent overlaps or gaps in service. With the special needs child, there often are a large number of services, treatments, and variety of providers involved – which can serve to overwhelm families.

The community health nurse, working as a case manager for the child and family, can facilitate regular meetings of all healthcare providers involved with the case, identify when new services are required, help assure quality of care along a continuum of services, and decrease the fragmentation of care that might otherwise exist (Public Health Nursing Section, 2001).

A model of case management often found in public health is that of the *interdisciplinary team*, where each discipline involved with the child's care is represented on the team (examples include social work, speech therapy, physical therapy, and nursing). Nurses can assist personnel in other healthcare or educational disciplines to understand the implication of the conditions causing the child's special needs, and how these special needs may require adaptations to individualized educational plans (IEPs), or the individualized family service plan (IFSP) (Davis & Steele, 1991).

Although all members contribute to the development of a comprehensive plan of care, one member of this team is designated as "lead" or "primary"

PUBLIC HEALTH AND SCHOOL HEALTH NURSING

to assure that this plan is implemented in the agreed-upon manner. It is also important that this "lead" or "primary" member has a clear understanding of the needs, questions, desires, and worries of the whole family, as well as the needs of the individual child.

In addition, it is crucial that all members of the interdisciplinary team have a clear understanding of the multiple and complex array of services that may involved with the child's care. These may include systems such as:

> *early intervention (EI) and special education services (mandated by the Individual with Disabilities Act), maternal and child services for children with special health needs (mandated by Title V of the Social Security Act), income support benefits (mandated by the Supplemental Security Income provision of the Social Security Act), state funded services through such agencies as the Departments of Mental Health or Mental Retardation and Developmental Disabilities, and publicly provided (e.g. Medicaid) or privately purchased health care services.(Krauss, Wells, Gulley, & Anderson, 2001, p. 166)*

There is a clear link between activities designed to assist the special needs child and family so that the child can be maintained in the home, and the *Healthy People 2010* objective 6–7: to reduce the number of people with disabilities in congregate care facilities, consistent with permanency-planning principles, to 0 by 2010 (US Department of Health and Human Services, 2000). Providers functioning in the case manager role need to be knowledgeable about the services available to the family, conversant with the complex governmental systems governing entitlement programs, and sensitive to the family's need for emotional, social, and financial support (Ardito, Botuch, Freeman, & Levy, 1997).

A guiding principle is that case managers seek to optimize the self-care capabilities of individuals and families, and the capacity of the systems and communities surrounding this child/family unit, in order to coordinate and provide services (Public Health Nursing Section, 2001). Case managers should not be viewed as a "solution" to the complexity of services and resources surrounding the family and child, but rather as a facilitator who will work with families to help map out appropriate routes to the desired destination (Krauss et al., 2001).

An initial task for the case manager may be to help the family access services and resources for basic needs in order to strengthen the overall unit, while simultaneously building rapport and trust with the family (Ardito et al., 1997, p. 61). Contracting with the family in order to explore mutual expectations and understandings, and to define agreed-upon roles and boundaries, can offer mutual advantages to both the care provider and the family. Such a contract would make explicit what the professional is able to do, what the family could expect from the professional, what the family has to offer, and what the professional can expect of the family (Dale, 1996).

A linked concept to case management is that of *resource utilization*, Standard #14 for Public Health Nursing. When engaging in this process, the public health nurse should consider factors related to the safety, effectiveness, cost, and impact on practice and on the population of focus, in the planning and delivery of nursing and public health programs, policies, and services (American Nurses' Association, 2007b).

Implicit in this standard is the expectation that public health nurses engage in ongoing or "formative" evaluation of the effectiveness of each resource applied to, and the consequent modification or augmentation of intervention plans based on such evaluations. It is of limited or no use to link families and special needs children to programs that are inappropriate, ineffective, or poorly funded, or that have only limited means to participate fully in the interdisciplinary team process.

It is also of paramount importance that families are linked to programs that respect the family's own goals and wishes for their child. Ongoing assessment of the child with special needs also needs to be family-centered, focusing on the family's quality-of-life goals for the special needs child (Johnson et al., 2005). Listening actively to the family is a key element in the trust-building phase, which is a necessary prerequisite to any problem-solving (Dale, 1996).

National core outcomes for children with special health care needs (CSHCN) have been set by the federal Maternal and Child Health Bureau. These include:

- families of CSHCN will partner in decision making and will be satisfied with the services they receive

- CSHCN will received coordinated, ongoing comprehensive care within a medical home

- families of CSHCN will have adequate private and/or public insurance to pay for the services that they need

- children will be screened early and continuously for special healthcare needs

- community-based service systems will be organized so that families can use them easily, and

- youths with special healthcare needs will receive the services necessary to make transitions to adult life, including adult health care, work, and independence (McPherson et al., 2004).

Helping families become partners in decision making (Core Outcome #1) often includes multiple iterations of the problem-solving process. As described by Dale (1996), the following steps outline a problem-solving process used by public health nurses and other healthcare workers functioning in a case management role:

1. Work with the family to define the nature of the problem or dilemma

2. Look at various options to solve the problem, using a brainstorming technique

3. Gather and share information about alternative solutions

4. Examine the consequences of each proposed solution

5. Make a mutual decision on a solution or set of solutions

6. Develop an appropriate plan of action

7. Implement the plan/take action

8. Evaluate the adequacy of the decision in light of the feedback/evaluation

Taking an environmental or holistic view of the family requires case managers to involve the entire family, not just the CSHCN child and parents. The potential impact on unaffected siblings of a CSHCN child cannot be overlooked, nor can the impact on the family's relationship to the community at large, and on the parents' marital relationship (Dale, 1996).

Public health nurses and other healthcare professionals engaged in home visiting have a unique opportunity to assess the stress levels associated with these factors, and to work with families to devise workable solutions. The aspect of *case finding*, defined as locating individuals and families with identified risk factors and connecting them to resources (Public Health Nursing Section, 2001, p. 55), challenges nurses and other healthcare professionals involved with families to not overlook the needs of the non-CSHCN members of those families, and their possible risk factors for stress, illness, or need for respite.

EVIDENCE-BASED HOME VISITING PROGRAMS FOR CHILDREN WITH SPECIAL HEALTH NEEDS

Home visiting programs for families with young children "blossomed" after 1993, with the infusion of funding from federal and private sources (Gomby,

PUBLIC HEALTH AND SCHOOL
HEALTH NURSING

Culross & Behrman, 1999). However, despite widespread use of home visiting as a model for service delivery, scant research has been done on the content covered and processes used in home visiting of children with special healthcare needs, and how such visiting related to outcomes for the children and their families (McBride & Peterson, 1997). A survey of 193 nominated programs providing home visiting for children with special healthcare needs found that a major function of these home visits was to assist families in the coordination and integration of additional services needed from other agencies and resources (Roberts & Akers, 1996).

Home visiting for the CSHCN child and family is seen as a vehicle for delivery of a comprehensive array of early intervention services that are needed by the young child with disabilities, and his or her family (McBride & Peterson, 1997). For home visiting with both CSHCN and non-CSHCN populations, there is a focus on the importance of these early years and the pivotal role that parents play, in addition to the goal of improving the lives of children through encouraging changes in the attitudes, knowledge, and/or behavior of the parents (Gomby et al., 1999).

Home visiting may include the intervention of *health teaching*, which is defined in the Minnesota model of public health practice as the "communication of facts, ideas and skills that change knowledge, attitudes, values, beliefs, behaviors and practices and skills of individuals, families, systems and/or communities" (Public Health Nursing Section, 2001, p. 121). In the fast-developing sphere of social networking, parents may be encountering a dizzying array of information, not all of which may be reliable. An emerging aspect of health education is helping parents and other family members to be *informed consumers of knowledge* – employing savvy and skill in navigating the vast array of sites, documents, and resources available in cyberspace. The public health nurse, working in partnership with the family, assists the family to develop the skills of lifelong learning, particularly as it relates to the care and nurturing of their CSHCN child.

A related concept is that of *counseling*, defined as the establishment of an interpersonal relationship between a public health nurse and a community, system, family, or individual, intended to increase or enhance the capacity for self-care and coping, and which engages at an emotional level (Public Health Nursing Section, 2001, p. 151). Public health nurses working with families via home visiting are often called upon to provide counseling activities, tempered with the need to empower families and increase their capacity for self-care. If the family's needs are being addressed via a multidisciplinary team approach, it is incumbent on the public health nurse to be fully aware of the other professionals' involvement with the family and child, and what interventions or initiatives are being implemented, so that overlap and working at cross-purposes can be avoided.

THE CHILD WITH SPECIAL NEEDS IN THE SCHOOL SETTING

Despite compulsory education laws in effect nationwide since 1918, the educational needs of children with special healthcare needs were not addressed at a national level until 1975 (Pardini, 2002). Public Law (PL) 94-142, the Education for All Handicapped Children Act passed in 1975, required public schools nationwide to provide students who have a wide range of disabilities (such as physical handicaps, mental retardation, speech, vision and language problems, emotional and learning disorders) with a "free appropriate education" in the "least restrictive environment" (Public Law 94-142, Nov. 29, 1975; Pardini). This law made education possible for half a million previously unserved severely handicapped children, redefined the role of parents in the education of the child, and refined the concept and practice of individualized instruction (Will, 1985). PL 94-142 was subsequently reauthorized in 1990 and 1997, and was renamed the "Individuals with Disabilities Education Act" or IDEA (Pardini, 2002).

The long path forward for education of children with special healthcare needs parallels in many ways the civil rights struggles and victories in the United States during the preceding decade of the 1960s. The 1954 *Brown v. Board of Education* decision and the civil rights movement of the 1960s helped pave the way for similar gains for those children with disabilities, and energized parental advocacy on behalf of their special needs children (Pardini, 2002).

In an early analysis of this legislation, done five years after the Act was passed, several provisions were identified that had implications for school nursing (Altschuld & Downhower, 1980). First, local educational systems had to strive to develop mechanisms to identify all handicapped individuals from 3 to 21 years of age, and systematically include them in the public school system. This not only expanded the population of students the school nurses would be expected to care for, but also vastly increased the complexity and challenges imposed by a variety of handicaps found in this new population of CSHCN. In addition, this Act expanded the age range of those considered to be within the educational system, so that children as young as 3 years of age, and as old as 21 years of age, would still be eligible for participation in the school system.

Second, there were training needs implied in the Act, both for teachers and all ancillary school staff, as well as for the school nurses themselves. Some states, such as Pennsylvania, have specified student-to-school nurse ratios built into their Public School Codes (Pennsylvania's code dated from 1965, at which time a ratio of 1500 students per nurse was mandated). The many additional duties and procedures added to the school nurse's role led the PA State Nurses Association to adopt a position that there should be a certified school nurse in every school, with a ratio of no higher than 750 students per certified nurse.

This is congruent with the American Nurses Association's position statement on school nursing, stating that the total number of students that a nurse serves should not exceed 750 (2007a). In addition, the Pennsylvania position stated that with increases in the population of special needs children, that ratio would decrease in proportion. For mainstreamed students, the ratio would be 225 students to one nurse; for special needs student populations requiring daily professional school nursing services or intervention, or dealing with severely or profoundly handicapped students, that ratio would decline to one certified school nurse for every 125 students (PA State Nurses Association, n.d.).

School nurses assume many of the same roles and functions as described in the prior section on public health nurses, including assessment, counseling, case management, and advocacy. Some school districts incorporate aspects of healthcare delivery within the union contract. For example, in the Spokane, Washington District 81 contract under Article A (student assistance/nursing specialists/truancy liaison), "school nurses may, in consultation with an approval of the coordinator of health services, determine the need for contracted *licensed* care for students with medication and/or treatment needs which require *licensed* intervention during the school day or the school week" (Spokane School District No. 81, 2009).

Another provision of this legislation with implications for school nurses was the requirement that all children with special healthcare needs have an Individualized Education Program (IEP) developed, based on the principles of a least restrictive educational environment to the greatest extent feasible (Altschuld & Downhower, 1980). Nurses' input into the plan, such as assisting teachers and other school personnel to gain a better understanding of the scope of each child's functional ability, and how the demands of treatment might impact the educational environment, constitutes key and vital information for this process.

A 2002 Issue Brief from the National Association of School Nurses speaks to the school nurse role in helping school personnel monitor chronic health conditions, while seeing an expansion of scope of nursing practice in the areas of increasingly complex technology needed to provide up-to-date care for student clients. The school nurse also enacts roles in leadership for development of health policies and programs, while serving as a liaison between school personnel, family, community and health care providers (National Association of School Nurses).

As in public health, school health nurses are expected to deliver increasingly complex care to a growing diversity of children with special healthcare needs, at a time when federal, state, and local support is under siege due to economic downturns. Even though federal support was promised to defray 40% of the additional costs to educate students with disabilities, and even though such spending has risen from $1.3 billion in 1997 to $6.3 billion in 2001, the federal government has never paid more than 15% of the total costs (Pardini, 2002).

Adding to this dilemma is that students with disabilities are less likely than their nondisabled peers to be successful as based on a variety of educational and labor force measurements (Lipsky & Gartner, 1996, p. 770), and are thereby more likely to depend on governmental assistance as they enter the adult years, and are less likely to be contributing members of society via such mechanisms as payroll taxes. However, merely casting this situation in terms of cost/benefit ratios ignores the social justice antecedents for "education for all," in which the morality of denying such education based on the presence of a handicap became no longer tolerable to the U.S. society.

One way to stretch limited resources is to employ both a case management model and a partnership approach between parents and care providers. In both instances, cooperative agreements about who will provide what services can prevent confusion and overlap, and can help identify gaps in service needing attention. In working as a partner with the parents and family, school nurses can contribute to the formation of a caring community around each child with special needs. Under this model, parents can develop recognition of their shared interests in and responsibilities for their child as they work with school personnel to create better programs and opportunities for their children (Epstein, 1995).

School nurses are in a privileged position to observe children with special healthcare needs grow and develop over time. The school nurses' astute observations, coupled with their expertise and knowledge of the pediatric population (both nonhandicapped and those with special healthcare needs), makes them invaluable members of the school team working to deliver education to the CSHCN population. Partnering with parents, resources, and other healthcare providers allows school nurses to develop expert knowledge in workable solutions for the challenges posed by the care needs of these children.

CONCLUSION

In conclusion, both public health and school health realms of nursing practice are crucial for success in meeting the healthcare and educational needs of the CSHCN population and their families. The many roles of these nurses often overlap in such dimensions as *advocacy, screening, outreach, consultation, collaboration, counseling, and case management* (Public Health Nursing Section, 2001). Working with the family and CSHCN client in partnership and a "power with" (versus an authoritarian "power-over" stance) allows the public health nurse and the school health nurse to pursue the mutual goal of

PUBLIC HEALTH AND SCHOOL HEALTH NURSING

empowerment of the client and family. Case management and comprehensive planning (such as the IFSP and IEP), allow for careful use of resources while maintaining necessary educational and health goals.

As changing attitudes about the disabled evolve through legislation, nursing practice is challenged to stretch and evolve as well. The Affordable Care Act of 2010, currently in its initial stages of implementation, will prohibit discrimination against children with preexisting conditions, and may have significant positive impacts for the CSHCN population (Health care reform in action, n.d.). Emerging definitions of the CSHCN population that expand to include those children at risk for developing chronic physical, developmental, behavioral, or emotional conditions will also expand nurses' involvement in such areas as therapeutic services, family support services, specialized nursing services, and the acquisition and use of equipment and supplies (McPherson et al., 1998).

REFERENCES

About TitleV. (n.d.). Association of Maternal & Child Health Programs. Retrieved from http://www.amchp.org/abouttitlev/pages/default.aspx

Altschuld, J., & Downhower, S. (1980). Issues in evaluating the implementation of Public Law 94-142. *Educational Evaluation and Policy Analysis*, 2(4), 31–38.

American Nurses Association (March 16, 2007a). Assuring safe, high quality health care in pre-K through 12 educational settings. Retrieved from http://www.nursingworld.org/MainMenuCategories/Policy-Advocacy/Positions-and-Resolutions/ANAPositionStatements/Position-Statements-Alphabetically/Assuring-Safe-High-Quality-Health-Care-in-Pre-K-Through-12-Educational-Settings.html

American Nurses' Association. (2007b). *Public health nursing: Scope and standards of practice*. Silver Spring, MD: Nurses' Books.org.

Ardito, M., Botuch, S., Freeman, S., & Levy, J., 1997. Delivering home-based case management to families with children with mental retardation and developmental disabilities. *Journal of Case Management*, 6(2), 56–61.

Center for Children with Special Needs (n.d.). Introduction to care coordination. Retrieved from http://cshcn.org/planning-record-keeping/what-care-coordination

Dale, N. (1996). *Working with families of children with special needs: Partnership and practice*. New York, NY: Routledge.

Davis, B., & Steele, S. (1991). Case management for young children with special health care needs. *Pediatric Nursing*, 17(1), 15–19.

Epstein, J. (1005). School/family/community partnerships: Caring for the children we share. *Phi Delta Kappan*, 76(9), 701–719.

Family Village (n.d.). A global community of disability-related resources. Retrieved from http://www.familyvillage.wisc.edu/

Gomby, D., Culross, P., & Behrman, R. (1999). Home visiting: Recent program evaluations – Analysis and recommendations. *The Future of Children*, 9(1), 4–26.

Health care reform in action (n.d.). The Affordable Care Act. Retrieved from http://www.whitehouse.gov/healthreform/healthcare-overview#healthcare-menu

PUBLIC HEALTH AND SCHOOL HEALTH NURSING

Johnson, C., Kastner, T., & the Committee/Section on Children with Disabilities (2005). Helping families raise children with special health care needs at home. *Pediatrics* *115*(2), 507–511.

Krauss, M., Wells, N., Gulley, S., & Anderson, B. (2001). Navigating systems of care: Results from a national survey of families of children with special health care needs. *Children's Services: Social Policy, Research, and Practice, 4*(4), 165–187.

Legislative History: 1935 Social Security Act. (n.d.). Retrieved from http://www .ssa.gov/history/35actinx.html

Lipsky, D., & Gartner, A. (1996). Inclusion, school restructuring, and the remaking of American society. *Harvard Educational Review, 66*(4), 762–796.

McBride, S., & Peterson, C. (1997). Home-based early intervention with families of children with disabilities: Who is doing what?. *Topics in Early Childhood Education, 17*(2), 209–234.

McPherson, M., Weissman, G., Strickland,B., et al. (2004). Implementing community-based systems of services for children and youths with special health care needs: How well are we doing?. *Pediatrics 113*(5), 1538–1544.

McPherson, M., Arango, P., Fox, H., et al. (1998). A new definition of children with special health care needs. *Pediatrics 102*(1), 137–139.

Mentro, A. (2003). Health care policy for medically fragile children. *Journal of Pediatric Nuring, 18*(4), 225–232.

Military Homefront (n.d.). Special Needs/EFMP Overview. Retrieved from http://www .militaryhomefront.dod.mil/portal/page/mhf/MHF/MH F_HOME_1?section_id=20 .40.500.570.0.0.0.0.0

National Association of School Nurses Issue Brief. (2002). School health nursing services role in health care: Role of the school nurse. Retrieved from http://www.nasn .org/Default.aspx?tabid=279

PA State Nurses Association (n.d.). Position statement on school nurse-to-student ratio. Retrieved from http://www.panurses.org/site/resources/Position/positions .cfm?action&ID=18

Pardini, P. (2002). The history of special education. *Rethinking Schools, 16*(3). Retrieved from http://www.rethinkingschools.org/archive/16_03/Hist163.shtml

Public Health Nursing Section. (2001). *Public health interventions: Applications for public health nursing practice*. St. Paul: Minnesota Department of Health.

Public Law 94–142 (S. 6); November 29, 1975. Education for All Handicapped Children Act of 1975; statement of findings and purpose. Retrieved from http://www .venturacountyselpa.com/Portals/45/Users/Public%2 0Law%2094.pdf

Roberts, R., & Akers, A. (1996). Family-level service coordination within home visiting programs. *Topics in Early Childhood Special Education, 16*(3), 279–301.

Spokane Regional Health District. (n.d.). Infant toddler network. Retrieved from http://www.srhd.org/services/itn.asp

Spokane School District No. 81 (2009). Collective bargaining agreement between Spokane School District No. 81 Board of Directors and the Spokane Education Association. Retrieved from http://www.nctq.org/docs/Spokane_CBA_09_12_ Certificated.pdf

Title V: Maternal and Child Health Services Block Grant Program, n.d.) Retrieved from: http://mchb.hrsa.gov/programs/titlevgrants/index.html

Understanding Title V of the Social Security Act. Health Resources and Services Administration, Maternal and Child Health Bureau. (n.d.). Retrieved from http://www .amchp.org/AboutTitleV/Documents/UnderstandingTitleV.pdf

PUBLIC HEALTH AND SCHOOL HEALTH NURSING

US Department of Health and Human Services. (2000). *Healthy people 2010* (2nd ed.). Washington, DC: US Government Printing Office.

Van Dyck, P., Kogan, M., McPherson, M., et al. (2004). Prevalence and characteristics of children with special health care needs. *Archives of Pediatric & Adolescent Medicine, 158*, 884–890.

Will, M. (1985). Educating children with learning problems: A shared responsibility. *Exceptional Children, 52*(5), 411–415.

END-OF-LIFE CARE FOR CHILDREN WITH SPECIAL NEEDS AND THEIR FAMILIES

Janet A. Lohan

Caring for Children with Special Healthcare Needs and Their Families: A Handbook for Healthcare Professionals, First Edition. Edited by Linda L. Eddy.

CHAPTER 12

END-OF-LIFE CARE
CHILDREN WITH SPECIAL NEEDS
AND THEIR FAMILIES

Healthcare professionals who care for children often prefer to think that children live in a carefree world where death never intrudes (Corr, 1996; Doka, 1996), and indeed that unhappiness of any sort should be far from a child's thoughts. However, this idealism is a highly unrealistic picture of childhood, and is a particularly unrealistic picture for children who live with the additional challenges of special needs. Children see that flowers that are picked soon wilt and lose their petals, autumn leaves turn color and fall from trees, garden vegetables stop growing after an autumn frost, bugs do not move after they are stepped on, goldfish sometimes are discovered floating on their backs in their goldfish bowls, and hamsters have a life expectancy of only 2–3 years. Given the statistics that nearly 2.5 million Americans die each year (Centers for Disease Control, 2010), a child may well experience the death of a grandparent, parent, sibling, friend, or peer before he or she reaches the age of 18. In addition, the fact that some conditions that children live with are life-limiting, protecting children from the realities of death and end-of-life issues, whether they involve the child him- or herself or someone the child knows and loves, is neither kind nor possible. Indeed, attempting to put a shield around a child leaves the child with the sense that death is such a horrible topic that it may never be discussed. This gives the child few opportunities to ask questions of the adults in his or her world and isolates the child from support and the chance to experience death as an opportunity to express both positive and negative emotions, learn coping skills, and gain a more mature understanding of both life and death.

CHILDREN'S UNDERSTANDING OF DEATH

Children are actively engaged in making sense of who they are and how the world works from birth, and they seek to understand how they ought to interact with people and things in their environment. This is true of all children, though children with special needs may have additional challenges as they cope with sensory deficits, mobility difficulties, communication problems, or developmental delays as they learn to relate to the world. In order to understand how children may comprehend the idea that living things (including people) die, it is necessary to understand developmental concepts about children's cognition and the way that young children make sense of the world in general. Although Piaget's (1929) theory of cognitive stages may be useful to understand the way that children think, this theory has problems when it comes to children's concepts of death. Moreover, children with special needs may or may not develop their thinking in the same ways that other children without special needs do, so Piaget's theory may not be the best framework to use to understand the way that children understand the concept of death. Corr (2008) and Speece and Brent (1996) reviewed literature about children's understanding of death and concluded that there are four main components to a mature concept of death. Caregivers who understand these components when explaining death to children will have a better understanding of why children do or do not understand death as adults do. The implications for children who do not yet understand the components are important for caregivers in their work with children whether or not a child has special needs.

Corr (2008) identified finality and universality as two central components of the concept of death. Finality, according to Corr, encompasses two elements: irreversibility and nonfunctionality.

> Irreversibility *means that the natural processes involved in the transition from being alive to being dead, as well as the state that results from these processes, cannot be reversed. Once the physical body of a living thing is dead, it can never be alive again (p. 11).*

Questions that researchers have used to assess children's understanding of irreversibility include "Can a dead person become alive again?", "What happens after you die?", "Can you come back to life after you die?", "If I gave some medicine to a dead person, could he become alive again?", "How do you make a dead thing come back to life?", and "How long will my friend's parent stay dead?" (Speece & Brent, 1996, pp. 34–35). These questions might also be used by a caregiver to assess a child's understanding of the irreversibility of death, although the question about "what happens after you die?" may be a question about physical changes in a dead body or a much larger spiritual question, so that "What happens to a body after it dies?" might be a more focused question to use. Again, it is important for a caregiver attempting to assess what a child knows to be sensitive to a child's individual and unique understanding ability, not chronological age or special need issues.

Younger children, in general, have more difficulty understanding irreversibility than do older children. Younger children are more likely to see death as a temporary and reversible condition; like sleep from which you might wake up or like a trip from which you might return. Children have identified such "interventions" to reverse death as eating or drinking, wishful thinking, praying, magical or medical intervention, or even spontaneous recovery (Speece & Brent, 1996). The idea of medical intervention being able to reverse death is difficult for children not to believe, given that many adults believe that CPR is a rather magical intervention to "bring someone back". However, the statistics about CPR as a lifesaving measure are not encouraging. The American Heart Association (AHA) reported in 2005 that, of 400,000 to 460,000 persons in the United States who experienced sudden cardiac arrest, only 2/3 received resuscitation attempts. Of those persons treated by Emergency Medical Services (EMS) after sudden cardiac arrest, 5–10% survive, and if the person was in ventricular fibrillation when treated by EMS, 15% survive to hospital discharge. If a person experiences sudden cardiac arrest in a hospital, only 17% survive to hospital discharge (American Heart Association, 2005). Clearly, though CPR can be a lifesaving intervention for a very few fortunate people, it is not the magical "returning the dead to life" intervention that a child (or an adult care provider) might realistically believe would invariably work.

Corr (2008) cited the second key element of finality as nonfunctionality: "that means the complete and absolute cessation of all the life-defining or functional capabilities (whether external and observable or internal and inferred) typically attributed to a living physical body" (p. 12). The key elements of finality are narrowly applied to only the physical body of the person, and leave open the question of some type of spiritual afterlife, resurrection, or reincarnation. This may be an important distinction for children who are taught a particular spiritual belief or value system.

Younger children have more difficulty grasping this element than do older children. They are more likely to think that dead bodies may somehow continue to have some physical functions after death. Kane, in a 1979 study, distinguished between external, readily observable functions such as eating and speaking and internal, inferred functions such as dreaming and knowing. She found that at any given age, it is easier for children to understand that external functions cease at death than for them to understand that internal functions cease at death as well.

Questions that Speece and Brent (1996) cited from research about nonfunctionality include "Can a dead person still hear?", "What happens after death?", "Is there anything a dead person can do?" and "Are people different after they die?". Again, the question about "What happens after death?" is one that could be viewed as either a question about physical nonfunctionality or one about spiritual continuation. A caregiver might use the question about whether there are things a dead person can still do to assess a child's understanding about the loss of function that dead bodies have.

Another aspect of the concept of death is *universality* (Corr, 2008). Corr explained that universality "brings together three closely related notions: all-inclusiveness, inevitability, and unpredictability" (p. 12).

All-inclusiveness refers to the child's understanding that *all* living things will eventually die. The understanding here is whether a person believes that all living things die, or does the person think there are exceptions and individuals who are somehow exempt from dying? Inevitability, in Corr's (2008) view, is linked to the all-inclusive concept in that "death is unavoidable for all living things . . . not merely to the extent or number of those who will die, but . . . none of them can escape their deaths. A person may avoid this or that death-related event, but not death itself" (p. 12). If a child believes that death is all-inclusive and inevitable, he or she might also believe that its timing might therefore be predictable and certain, but Corr stated that "in fact, death is *unpredictable* – anyone might die at any time" (p. 12) regardless of the person's circumstances or age. The question of when a particular person might die remains an open one for the person who understands this concept, and is presumably an open question for healthcare providers, who are notoriously inaccurate at predicting when a patient might die. This causes considerable happy confusion to people who have been told they have six months to live but who are indeed alive five years later, or great unhappiness to families who are told a person may have a year to live but then the person dies within a few days.

Speece and Brent (1996) asserted that younger children, in general, are more likely than older children to believe that death is not universal. Researchers have found that the exceptions that younger children cite include the child himself/herself, children in general, the child's immediate family members, teachers, and even the researchers asking children questions about the universality of death. Children have told researchers that if you are clever or lucky, you might not die, and in any case death is a remote future event. Evidence exists that children are likely to understand that they themselves will die before they understand that all other people will someday die. Younger children who believe in the remote future death idea are probably right, but this also means that they have not grasped the idea of the unpredictability of death (Speece and Brent). This may help to explain why young children might be less aware of the implications of dangerous behaviors; in addition to limitations in their thinking about cause-and-effect relationships, they are also not thinking about the risk of death in a dangerous situation.

Questions that researchers have used to assess children's understanding of the concept of universality could also be useful to the healthcare provider working with a child with special needs to assess a particular child's ability to understand the concept. Speece and Brent (1996) cited a number of questions, including "Will everybody die someday?", "Will you die someday?", "Do children ever die?", "When do people die?", "When will you die?", "Can we stop a person from dying?", and "Is there something I can do so that I won't ever die?". These questions could be used by a caregiver (though perhaps not all at once!) to bring up the topic of death and to assess what a particular child's understanding might be of the universality component. It is the child's level of understanding that is important, not the child's chronological age or developmental level. This level of understanding is particularly important to assess with a child with special needs; the caregiver must assess what the child is able to understand and neither overestimate nor underestimate the child's abilities either because of the child's special needs or in spite of those needs.

The fourth component of the concept of death is causality. Speece and Brent (1996) cited considerable difficulty in finding consensus among researchers as to this component, but they suggested that

the mature understanding of causality involves an abstract and realistic understanding of the external and internal events that might possibly cause an individual's death. This understanding is "abstract" in the sense that the causes specified are not restricted to particular individuals or events, but are classes of causes that are applicable to living things in general. It is "realistic" in the sense that the causes specified are generally accepted by mature adults as valid causes of death (pp. 36–37).

Younger children are more likely to describe unrealistic causes of death or specific concrete causes of death than are older children; researchers have found that younger children may believe that bad behavior causes death or guns or poison cause death. They focus more on external causes of death such as violence or accidents than internal causes of death such as illness or advanced age (Speece & Brent, 1996). This focus on external causality makes sense given the younger child's problems in understanding how the internal organs of the body work, because the child is unable to see them. Younger children often lack understanding that what ultimately causes death is a failure of one or more internal body systems or organs. If a young child does not know where a kidney is in the body or how it works, renal failure as a cause of death cannot make sense. It is important to understand that younger children may attribute bad behavior to causality; if a child has behaved badly in his or her own estimation and then a significant person dies, the child may feel very guilty for causing the death. By the same token, if a child believes that bad behavior causes death, he or she may work extremely hard to behave in positive ways to either make up for causing someone's death or to prevent future deaths. Believing that one's behavior can cause or prevent death is a large burden for a child to carry, and reassurance that this is not true may be a huge relief to a child who has been thinking this way.

Questions to assess children's understanding of causality include "Why do people die?" as a general question, "How can you die?" to focus on specific causes of death, and "Can people die because they were bad?" as a specific hypothetical cause. The question of "Why do people die?" could be construed as a physical causality question, or as a question with much larger spiritual overtones, so this question needs to be used cautiously to assess exactly what the caregiver is getting at with the child's understanding. The question of death by bad behavior could be used to refer to the dying person's behavior, and also to question a child about thinking that his or hertheir own behavior caused another person's death.

Speece and Brent (1996) became interested in a fifth component of the concept of death that seemed to be related to the components of irreversibility and nonfunctionality, but which differed in that, when adults were asked about the death of the physical body, some raised the possibility of some sort of "noncorporeal personal continuation after death" (p. 41). Different researchers have dealt with aspects of this noncorporeal continuation in various ways, and Speece and Brent, in their review of those studies, concluded that more research is needed to explore this concept further. Speece and Brent called for additional research about the way that children begin to develop a sense of noncorporeal continuation, and suggested that

> ... *the development of the conceptualization of noncorporeal continuation should be studied as a separate component in its own right. The appropriate methodology for exploring children's understandings about nonnaturalistic aspects of death, as separate from their understandings of the irreversibility and nonfunctionality of physical death, remains an interesting challenge (p. 42).*

Corr (2008) discussed this notion of continuation leading to questions by the child about what happens after death (not referring to the physical body) and what happens to the soul or spirit of a person after death. Corr stated that this questioning goes beyond the child's knowledge about finality, universality, and causality and reflects a conviction about some form of noncorporeal continuation:

> *The conviction may be expressed in various ways, such as a belief in the ongoing life of a soul in heaven without the body or the reincarnation of a soul in a new and different body. Various religious, philosophical, and spiritual systems have attempted to provide frameworks for these questions. The important point here is that many children try to carry their understandings beyond the death of the physical body (p. 13).*

The significant point of this noncorporeal continuation idea is that the caregiver of a child must understand the framework that the family is using to understand the "what happens next?" questions, so that the family's spiritual system is supported and the child is not confused by the caregiver's injecting of his or her spiritual beliefs into the situation if those beliefs contrast with the family's beliefs and values.

A significant challenge in doing research about the component of noncorporeal continuation is accounting for different spiritual and faith community beliefs about an afterlife, reincarnation, or resurrection possibility as taught by different spiritual traditions. It is not enough for a caregiver who is assessing a child's understanding of death to ask the questions about irreversibility and nonfunctionality to children who are being taught a spiritual message that they should await a soul reunion with a dead person in heaven, or that the soul will be reincarnated into another body in the quest for nirvana, or that physical bodies will be resurrected for a Last Judgment at some future time.

It is important for a caregiver to be able to assess what a child understands about what has happened to a person the child cares about who is either dying or who has already died. Although Speece and Brent (1996) suggested that advancing age increased a child's ability to understand the components of death, cognitive development is "only helpful and contributory rather than necessary" (p. 44) in helping the child develop a more adult concept of death. Other characteristics that may affect a child's thinking about the concept of death include culture, death-related experiences, intelligence, and having a life-threatening illness. However, the research evidence is not yet clear about exactly how different characteristics affect a child's understanding. The concern of the caregiver here is what a child understands and how to explain to a child a death that is happening now, given the child's current level of thinking. It is important for caregivers to assess what is going on with the child's thinking, be available to answer the child's questions, and support the child as he or she struggles with new understandings that death is universal and irreversible, that the body is nonfunctional, and that death has had a physiological cause. In addition, the caregiver needs to support the family's beliefs and values about spiritual aspects of noncorporeal continuation so that the child's spiritual needs are met.

Corr (2008) described the caregiver's role with young children thus:

The basic lesson . . . is twofold: (1) Children do make an effort to grasp or understand death when it comes into their lives; and (2) a good way – perhaps the only effective way – to gain insight into a child's understandings of death is to establish a relationship of confidence and trust with the child, and to listen carefully to the child's comments, questions, and concerns about loss and death (p. 14).

Talking to adolescents about the concept of death presents a caregiver with additional challenges. Balk (2008) discussed three developmental tasks that mark the adolescent's transition from adolescence to adulthood as gaining skill and competence to "(1) make career choices, (2) enter into and maintain intimate relationships, (3) form an autonomous identity. In short, the developmental tasks adolescents are expected to master involve responsibility, interpersonal intimacy, and individuality" (p. 26). Although by adolescence a person may have an understanding of the components of universality, nonfunctionality, and irreversibility, Noppe and Noppe (1996) contended that there are developmental issues in adolescence that make a mature understanding of these components difficult for the adolescent to truly grasp. Universality bumps into adolescent participation in high-risk activities such as street racing or rock climbing. Yes, the adolescent knows that everyone dies, but somehow that principle does not quite apply to *this* adolescent *now*. Corr (1996) cited the adolescent's needs to become independent of parents, cope with frustration, and get approval from peers as strong motivators to take risks despite the knowledge that risky behaviors are hazardous (for *other* people!). This idea may be significant for the adolescent with special needs; caregivers must remember that the motivation to get peer acceptance is a strong one for all adolescents, and that those with special needs who do not want to be seen as different from healthy peers may be tempted to go to great lengths to get approval and acceptance from a peer group. These lengths might include risky behaviors – and the adolescent with special needs may be more at risk in doing some things because of his or her special needs than would be an adolescent without those limitations. In addition, Noppe and Noppe stated that nonfunctionality and irreversibility might not be serious concerns for an adolescent who can now consider alternatives. "Fascination with various alternatives to a permanent and total ending of life – an antimatter universe, an afterlife, reincarnation, and so forth" (p. 26) may offer the adolescent possibilities for some sort of parallel functioning. These alternatives, however, may be intriguing for an adolescent to ponder but would be cold comfort to bereaved family members left behind (Noppe and Noppe).

Adolescents are faced with an array of difficulties as they cope with the developmental challenges of adolescence and also try to understand death as a concept:

> There are strong biological tensions between physical and sexual maturation, which also herald inevitable decline. A rich, cognitive explosion is found in young, logical minds that must also contemplate their own demise. Social conflicts among friends, between adults and peers, and among competing or diverse cultural pressures may introduce an increased sense of isolation. An emotional "roller coaster" of reworking attachment relationships, and the emerging sense of personal identity, contrasts with feelings of anxiety, depression and the loss of self (Noppe and Noppe, 1996, p. 26).

The adolescent who has special needs is in a particularly painful place in terms of these conflicts. How does the special need affect physical and sexual maturation? Will the adolescent with special needs be attractive to a sexual partner, and will the adolescent be prepared to deal with the consequences of sexual behavior (physical, social, and emotional – might the adolescent be manipulated, exploited, or hurt by another person)? How does the special need affect the adolescent's cognition and ability to understand situations that may be risky? What is the effect of the special need on the adolescent's social life and the person's ability to relate to peers and be accepted by them? What is the effect of the adolescent's special need on family relationships – is the adolescent still dependent on parents as a care recipient, and, if so, how does that influence the adolescent's ability to differentiate the self from others? Adding on the ideas of death – and death as a very real personal possibility due to the effects of the special need – places this adolescent in a very difficult position as he or she faces adolescent transitions such as attending middle school or high school, and medical care moves from pediatric to adult care settings.

END-OF-LIFE CARE FOR CHILDREN WITH SPECIAL NEEDS AND THEIR FAMILIES

DIFFICULT CONVERSATIONS ABOUT DEATH AND DYING WITH CHILDREN AND THEIR FAMILIES

Now that it is more clear what children are thinking and understanding about death as a complex concept, caregivers are still faced with difficult questions about "What do I say to a child in my care about the death of a person the child cares about?" and, even more problematic, "What do I say to a child in my care about the child's impending death?" The question remains as to whether the caregiver's intent ought to be to push a child into a more mature understanding than he or she currently has. Would increasing a child's understanding be helpful for a young child, or would it just increase a child's anxiety to think about someone being "dead forever" and having everyone in the child's world be subject to an unpredictable and inevitable death when the child is very dependent on the care of adults to survive? Must a child know, and be reminded, that a dead parent is "never coming back," or is it harmful to think that the dead parent may somehow come back for a visit, only for the child to be disappointed when that visit never happens? Are there things we might say to the dying child that would increase a child's anxiety, and others that would decrease that anxiety? What should the caregiver say? What should the caregiver *not* say? Wishing to spare a child pain is a caregiver's responsibility, and the very definition of "giving care" includes physical and emotional comfort and support. Because it is obviously not possible to deny the reality of death in a child's world, how could a caregiver initiate a conversation with a child, or respond to a child who initiates a conversation?

Rabbi Earl Grollman (1995) described a gentle, caring way to inform a child about a death of another person. He began by saying that "*What* is said is significant, but how it is said will have a greater bearing on whether youngsters develop unnecessary fears or will be able to accept, within their abilities, the reality of death" (p. 20). Rabbi Grollman emphasized using warmth, kindness, and affection in the approach to the child, as well as assuring that accurate information is given. Giving the child the opportunity to talk and ask questions is important. If the child changes the subject or goes out to play, it is the child's way of saying that the information is overwhelming and disturbing, and that the child cannot deal with news all at once (Grollman).

Grollman (1995) also listed a number of possible reactions that children may have to the news that someone has died: denial, bodily distress, hostile reactions to the deceased, idealization, panic, and guilt (pp. 21–22). These reactions are normal for children, and Grollman suggested that the child's school or day care center be informed of the death so that teachers will be aware of behavior changes in the child and the reason for those changes. He also listed danger signals that caregivers must watch for; if after several months children continue to:

- Look sad all the time and experience prolonged depression

- Keep up a hectic pace and cannot relax the way they used to with you and their friends

- Not care about how they dress and look

- Seem tired, or unable to sleep, with their health suffering markedly

- Avoid social activities and wish to be alone more and more

- Be indifferent to school and hobbies they once enjoyed

- Experience feelings of worthlessness and self-incrimination

- Rely on drugs and/or alcohol

- Let their moods control them instead of controlling their moods (p. 26)

These symptoms should prompt parents and caregivers to consider a referral to a professional for help. Grollman stressed that seeking professional advice is not a weakness, but instead demonstrates strength and love for a grieving child who is struggling.

Several authors have written about strategies to use to discuss a life-threatening illness with children. Again, it is important to consider the child's developmental level and to take into account a child's strengths and limitations. These conversations are not easy for adults to have, and the distress is compounded when the ill person is a child. However, there are strategies available so that children are not left without support and love during the last months, weeks, or days of their lives.

Beale, Baile, and Aaron (2005) suggested the use of the "6 Es" strategy as a guide to communicating with dying children and their families:

Establish an agreement with parents, children, and caregivers early on the relationship with them concerning open communication. Begin by exploring the attitudes of the child's caregivers about sharing medical information with the child and answering any concerns they might have ... Engage the child at the opportune time. A newly diagnosed serious illness, or the occasion when a child takes a turn for the worse, are medical events that should trigger discussion ... Explore what the child already knows and wants to *know about the illness. It is often surprising how much information the child already has and the extent of his or her fantasies and concerns ... **Explain** medical information according to the child's needs and age. Children often have questions about what is happening and what is going to happen to them ... **Empathize** with the child's emotional reactions. Allowing a child to be upset and express feelings while the caregivers provide physical contact may be painful for the caregivers. Nonetheless, once emotions are vented, discussions of more concrete concerns often follows ... **Encourage** the child by reassuring him or her that you will be there to listen and to be supportive. Isolation and anxiety about his or her support system and about symptoms such as pain are prime concerns for children who are dying. Acknowledging the fact that cure is not possible but that life's tasks can continue, even if only in a limited way, provides some stability to the family and is perceived as a hopeful attitude (p. 3631).*

Although the "6 Es" strategy focuses on children with cancer, the technique could also be applied to other disease processes that are life-limiting for children. What this strategy can do is decrease the child's uncertainty, which can be an issue for children given their lack of capacity to get information that can be reassuring. Beale, Baile, and Aaron (2005) stressed that caregivers must acknowledge their own emotional pain so that it does not become a barrier to open communication. Avoidance of the discussion of dying out of concern for not frightening or depressing a child is counterproductive and leaves the child unsupported, anxious, and isolated (Beale, Baile, and Aaron).

Doka (1996) described two significant differences between the adult who is faced with a life-threatening illness and a child who is affected. Information and communication were the first difference, and developmental issues related to childhood were the second.

Doka pointed to the work of various authors (Bluebond-Langner, 1978; Doka, 1982; Gunther, 1949) who asserted that attempts to protect a child from any knowledge of death, including evading a child's questions, were counterproductive. Doka (1996) cited four dimensions to the child's experience that make protection impossible:

First, in various ways children can acquire a tremendous degree of medical sophistication ... Second, children often have external cues concerning their own health situation. They can sense the anxieties and concerns around them ... Third, often their peers are effective sources of information for children ... Finally, children respond to their own internal cues. They know they are in pain; they can sense when they are weaker and sicker (pp. 96–97).

Doka (1996) listed three primary questions that should guide caregivers who are deciding how to communicate or share information about a life-threatening

END-OF-LIFE CARE FOR CHILDREN WITH SPECIAL NEEDS AND THEIR FAMILIES

illness with a child: "What does a child need to know?", "What does a child want to know?", and "What can a child understand?" The question of what a child needs to know is important, in Doka's view, if the child is to be able to participate and have a sense of control during the illness. Differences in illnesses, age, and personality need to be taken into account. The timing of information is important; at the time of diagnosis, it is perhaps not appropriate to discuss all of the long-term potential effects of an illness, but Doka stressed that immediate and short-term implications need to be discussed so that the child can participate in the treatment plan. Also, the child needs to know what treatments are planned and what side effects might happen, in an honest way. Clichéd reassurances that "everything will be okay" are not helpful; a life-limiting illness will not be "okay," and the child will learn not to trust the information he or she is given, leading to reduction in anxiety now but a resurgence of anxiety later in an atmosphere of distrust. Doka asserted that "honest and hopeful responses, such as 'we are doing all we can' are both truthful and reassuring" (p. 98). An important issue for caregivers to remember is that there is never a time when "there is nothing more that we can do." There is *always* something more to do: being with the child; offering care, support, pain management, and touch as appropriate, and respite for families, is not "nothing" from either the caregiver's perspective or the child's.

In Doka's view, the second question of "What does a child want to know?" is also important. He stressed the importance of recognizing that what a child asks about is what the child is ready to hear. However, a key point is to really understand what a question means before jumping into a response. It may be that the child is asking for information, reassurance, or both (Doka, 1996). Remember that the young child is likely to be unclear about cause and effect in his or her ideas about death, and may think that he or she may be guilty of wrongdoing that has led to his or her own illness or the illness of another person. Also, it is not enough to reassure the child once, and it may take several reassurances to persuade a child that his or her actions did not cause an illness to happen. This point may be particularly salient for the child with special needs to know that nothing the child did led to his or her condition.

The third question is "What can a child understand?" This question is particularly applicable to children with special needs. Some special needs limit a child's mobility, which may be an effect of illness as well. Others limit a child's perception of the world, which may also be an effect of illness. Still others may limit a child's ability to understand and make sense of the world, and this may also be an effect of illness. Some conditions inhibit a child's ability to interact socially with others and read and interpret verbal and nonverbal cues from others. Doka (1996) explained that caregivers need to take the child's understanding into account. "As children grow and develop, they differ in their vocabulary, sense of cause and effect, presence or absence of magical thinking, and ability to understand abstract thoughts" (p. 99).

Developmental issues related to childhood are the second component that Doka (1996) cited as significant when discussing a life-limiting illness with a child:

> *A child's entire experience of illness will be greatly affected by his or her developmental level. At each point in development, a child's own developmental level will influence both how the child responds to illness and how the experience with illness may affect subsequent development (p. 99).*

Infants have, in Doka's view, particular problems with serious illness and treatment regimens. Periods of separation from parents; the changing environments of a hospital, outpatient clinic, and home; and painful medical procedures about which the infant has no say can all negatively affect the child-parent attachment process and the infant's sense of trust in the parent to meet his or her needs (Doka, 1996). When a parent stands by and allows a painful medical procedure to occur, an infant learns both that the parent is not trustworthy and that medical personnel are hurtful. Doka pointed out that as the infant moves into toddlerhood, physical constraints on the child caused either by the illness or treatments for the illness, as well as parental overprotectiveness that may result from the parent's fear about losing the child, interfere with the development of the autonomy so integral to the healthy toddler's sense of self, and limit the child's normal ability to explore the world as a healthy toddler would. Parents, who are understandably worried and fearful given the diagnosis of a life-limiting problem in a very young child, may not set appropriate limits on the toddler's behavior or may be inconsistent in their discipline of a toddler based on their view of how sick the toddler is; these approaches do not teach the child appropriate boundaries and limits (Doka, 1996). This lack of limits can quickly lead to a "more terrible two": a toddler who is without respect for others and very unhappy with him- or herself, as well as the toddler lives within changing boundaries and unclear restraints on his or her behavior. As the child with an illness moves into middle childhood, Doka stated that additional challenges present themselves. The addition of the demands of school causes a number of problems for the child:

> *First, intermittent outbreaks of disease and side effects of treatment may impair academic performance. Second, the treatment regimen may be difficult to manage within the school environment. Third, schools unwittingly thrust ill children into interactions with healthy peers. In some cases, this may be positive, reinforcing a sense of normalcy for the child. In other cases, such confrontations may create difficulties. Interactions with other children may accentuate the ill child's sense of differentness. Or peers may share troubling information about the disease with an ill child (p. 100).*

Doka suggested that a child with a serious illness might benefit academically from special education classes. There are positive and negative aspects to a special education classroom for a child with a serious illness. The child can receive an individualized education plan (IEP) that could account for frequent absences and unclear thinking that may accompany medical treatments. However, placement in special education may lead to stigma and impair the child's self-esteem. Special education might also isolate the child from healthy peers and limit the social support the child could receive from being mainstreamed in a regular classroom (Doka, 1996). In an atmosphere of high-stakes testing and evaluation of academic performance that are linked to school funding, a child's ability to perform well in school is important. A child who already has special needs may need a modification of the IEP to take into account an illness in addition to whatever special needs with which the child was already coping, such as a child with Down's Syndrome who is diagnosed with leukemia as well.

Doka expressed the issues of the child coping with a life-limiting illness during middle childhood:

> *During this stage of development, the key developmental tasks of mastery and independence may be complicated by the illness. Here, too, the overprotectiveness of parents and the physical constraints of the illness can impair the search for mastery. Yet this quest for maturity can also be effectively employed in coping with the illness. By extending to the child an active role in adhering to a treatment regimen and by giving the child a measure of control in treatment decisions, a sense of mastery can be developed and the child's effective coping with the illness strengthened. Youngsters in childhood often possess two other notable strengths. First, they are usually able to accept the help of supportive adults, something they may be more reluctant to do in adolescence. Second, often they can also draw strength and comfort from their philosophical or religious beliefs (p. 100).*

One of the things that caregivers must think about as they care for schoolage children with special needs includes the amount of time that these children spend in the company of adults. Although healthy children spend time with adults such as parents, teachers, sports coaches, and perhaps music or dance teachers, children with special needs may spend much more time with parents as they receive care from them, and also may interact with physicians, nurses, physical and occupational therapists, or speech therapists. Adding an illness into the mix will increase the time spent with adults as well. Although these adults are important in the child's care, it is also important for a middle childhood child to have contact with peers and siblings too. Although some activities of healthy childhood will not be possible for a child coping with the limitations imposed by an illness, having a friend to "hang out with" who does not see the medical equipment or treatments but just sees the child as a person is helpful beyond measure to a child. The friend learns to deal with the differences between him- or herself and others, and the child with the illness learns that he or she is still acceptable and important to another child.

Adolescents who have been diagnosed with a life-threatening illness pose additional challenges for caregivers. Stevens and Dunsmore (1996) explained the reactions of adolescents to a life crisis:

> When a young person is in crisis or under threat, regression to a more concrete way of thinking often occurs. Frequently, adolescents are able to say the "right" thing and discuss complex issues with a maturity beyond their years, yet behave in a very different manner. Interruption of the developmental process by illness may interfere with the adolescent's developing abilities to perceive the future and to understand the consequences of behavior. Because cognitive development is so influenced by psychosocial maturity, the choices adolescents make may not be easily understood by adults (p. 108).

This difficulty with regression is exacerbated by the conflict between dependence and independence that a life-threatening illness causes. Although the adolescent may need to rely on parents for support during a crisis, they also want to spend time away from their parents associating with peers and confiding in those peers rather than in their parents. The healthy adolescent struggles with developmental tasks, social changes, and relationships with family and peers, and the adolescent with a life-threatening illness must cope with these struggles as well as the stresses brought on by the illness, its treatment demands, and the side effects of treatment (Stevens & Dunsmore, 1996).

When compared to younger children, it is even more important for adolescents to have information about the disease process with which they are dealing, involvement in the plan of treatment, and participation in the making of decisions about their care (Cassileth, Zupkis, Sutton-Smith, & March, 1980; Dunsmore & Quine, 1995). "Further, terminally ill adolescents are usually more concerned about how their family and friends will be affected by their death than about themselves. They are not so much afraid of death as of the dying" (Stevens & Dunsmore, 1996, p. 109).

A life-threatening illness sets an adolescent on a trajectory that includes a number of losses along the way. Among the losses cited by Stevens and Dunsmore (1996) are the former healthy self, the healthy body image, health itself, day-to-day school life, independence, relationships with parents, relationships with siblings, relationships with boyfriends or girlfriends, certainty about the future, indicators of the future, and changes in the sense of hope. Caregivers must be aware that these losses are happening in the life of the adolescent, and be prepared for the adolescent's reactions to these losses so that the caregiver can be supportive and helpful to the adolescent, and to the adolescent's family, to facilitate coping. Maintaining open, honest communication and the adolescent's sense of dignity and privacy despite changes due to the illness's progress are vitally important; in many ways the adolescent has the same developmental needs as healthy adolescents do, and living while in the process of dying is an important goal. It is a privilege to work with adolescents who have a life-threatening illness. "In confronting the possibility of death, and in dying, they teach us with humor and with love, about the preciousness of life and living" (Stevens & Dunsmore, 1996, p. 135).

PROVIDING CRISIS INTERVENTION FOR FAMILIES AND PEERS AFTER A CHILD DIES

What is a caregiver to do and say to survivors after the worst has happened? What help can he or she provide to those left behind when the child's life has been lost? One of the first tasks for the caregiver is to take care of him- or herself. Often this topic is listed last in a list of interventions, but in actuality it needs to be taken care of first, because if the caregiver is not intact and has not built a framework of self-care and support, there will be nothing left to give to the bereaved family. It is very draining to invest significant amounts of time and energy into caring for a child and then have that child die; a sense of personal failure can be a significant part of the caregiver's grief over the child's death. Unless the caregiver recognizes and acknowledges these feelings of grief and failure, it will be very difficult to be supportive of the child's family. As Davies et al. (1996) stated:

> *Nurses who work with children who die need to find meaning in their work that helps resolve their grief distress. Sharing the experience with other nurses offers the most support. When nurses tell their stories to empathetic colleagues, they review and resolve the struggle with each telling. When nurses use each other as listening posts, confidantes, confessors and teachers, they find ways to cope with caring for dying children. Opportunities for mentoring should be available to all nurses, especially to inexperienced nurses facing the care of a dying child for the first time. Flexibility in patient assignments, time away from the situation during the shift and after the death, and time off to attend the child's funeral all help nurses manage grief. Opportunities to brief, debrief, review and analyze the situation in a safe, supportive environment help nurses cope with current and subsequent stresses in their practice (p. 506).*

Caregivers must believe that they are entitled to feel the grief that invariably follows the death of a child in their care. This grief is described by Papadatou (2000) as "the private shadows experienced by health professionals who are exposed to multiple deaths of patients ... [t]heir private shadows comprise a wide range of painful experiences that remain hidden from public view, are often silent, and sometimes disregarded by professionals themselves" (p. 61). Papadatou cited six categories of losses that professionals experience in their role as health professionals:

1. Loss of a close relationship with a particular patient

2. Loss due to professional's identification with the pain of family members

3. Loss of one's unmet goals and expectations and one's professional self-image and role

4. Losses related to one's personal system of beliefs and assumptions about life

5. Past unresolved losses or anticipated future losses

6. The death of self

pp. 62–63). Healthcare professionals need to attend to these multiple losses, which may happen over and over during the course of a career. Sometimes losses occur more than once in a single shift, on a daily basis, or at least weekly or monthly. One issue that is not recognized often enough is the dilemma of the caregiver who cares for a dying child until the death occurs, but then is interrupted by the needs of other living patients. How is the caregiver to leave the body of the dead child to answer a call light from another patient with mundane requests for ice chips, juice, or pain medication? This cognitive dissonance is unrecognized in the literature, but completely recognized by the caregiver trying to cope simultaneously with issues literally of life and death. Although caregivers may not feel the same loss that a family does when a child dies, the family only deals with one death while the caregiver must go on to deal with several other clients' needs, and deal with additional child deaths soon after the first death occurred, over and over again. Keene, Hutton, Hall and Rushton (2010) advocated the use of bereavement debriefing sessions for healthcare professionals to review the cases of children who have died, grief responses of caregivers, emotional responses, strategies for coping with grief, and lessons learned from caring for a particular child and family. Their research showed that the opportunity to express one's grief and reflect on caring for a particular patient and family allows healthcare professionals to learn to manage their own grief experience to continue to serve the many families who need their expertise and care (p. 189).

Once the caregiver's own needs are met, he or she can focus on the needs of the surviving family and peers, which are considerable and complex. Again, developmental considerations are extremely important when designing intervention strategies for survivors. Understanding what is happening with the

END-OF-LIFE CARE FOR CHILDREN WITH SPECIAL NEEDS AND THEIR FAMILIES

family and children who survive after a child's death is key to planning and implementing appropriate intervention strategies for those survivors.

Parents who have had a child die are in a unique position. First of all, there is no one word in the English language to describe them. It is clear who is meant by the term "orphan," "widow," or "widower," but there is no such term for parents whose child has died, apparently because such an occurrence is linguistically and socially unacceptable. The best that the literature has been able to do to describe such parents is the term "bereaved parents." It is necessary to understand the changes that parents encounter in becoming parents in order to comprehend what has been lost by them with the child's death. Klass (1988), in a classic work on parental grief, explained that parenting contains the elements of identification, differentiation, and competence:

Identification with the child creates an opportunity for the parent to relive his or her own life through the child's developmental stages ... The identification with the child also creates the possibility for the ambivalence within the parent's self to become an ambivalence within the relationship to the child (p. 5).

One of the psychological tasks of parenting is to counter identification, to separate the child from the self, and to hold the child as an individual distinct from the self. When the child is experienced as being distinct, then the parent empathizes with the child and tries to meet the child's needs and desires on the child's terms rather than responding to the needs of and desires of the child as if they were the needs and desires of the parent (p. 6).

Part of the adult's sense of competence may be the ability to live up to the obligations of parenting bonds ... If adults do not feel competent in the parental role, they feel a sense of failure. They feel helpless and in panic (p. 7).

For parents, then, the death of a child challenges each of these elements. In addition, the child's death engenders "changes in the endocrine, immune, autonomic nervous, and cardiovascular systems" (Klass, 1988, p. 9) of the parent. These changes occur "simply because interaction with the child was one means by which the parent's hormonal balance was maintained" (p. 10). Two other significant, and long-lasting, characteristics are also true of parental grief, the characteristics of "(1) the loss of a part of the self and (2) the loss of a sense of competence and power" (p. 9).

Parents are therefore faced with the accomplishment of two very difficult tasks after the death of a child:

First, the parent must learn to live again in a world made poorer by the death of the child. That means not simply severing the tie with the child, but growing and changing the way one is in the world. The second task is retaining the bond with the child by internalizing the inner representation of the child in a way that brings solace (Klass, 1988, p. 17).

Bereaved parents find themselves forever changed by their child's death, and there seems to be a sense that "they are not the same person they were before the child's death" (Klass, 1988, p. 18). They have to restructure their sense of themselves and also the way that new self interacts with others in the social context surrounding them. Social support is crucial for all bereaved people, but bereaved parents in particular have a great deal of difficulty obtaining the level of social support that they need after the child's death:

While the parents strive to comprehend the reality of the loss, they find themselves within a social system that refuses to assimilate the truth that the child has died and that the parent has been wounded to the core of the self. The parents need to express feelings in order to understand and then to resolve the emotions that accompany the death of the child (p. 20).

These tasks are made all the more difficult if the parent has surviving children, who may resemble the dead child, and who continue to grow and develop, painful reminders of the ticking time that no longer includes the dead child. The dead child will not go off to kindergarten, get a driver's license, graduate from high school or college, find a life partner, have a career, and have children. Surviving children do these things, but not without varying degrees of difficulties, and yet the bereaved parent knows that whatever growth and development problems their surviving children have, they are at the very least alive to *have* problems. Enveloped in the own grief, parents have a great deal of difficulty empathizing with problems such as school bullies, acne, and getting a prom date when there is a shadow of the dead child who is not alive to have such problems – and who may have dealt with those problems, in the parent's estimation, much more effectively than the surviving children do.

The social context of the parents includes a world that does not have a word to describe them, and they represent, for other parents, a nightmare in that if one child can die, so could any child, or their child. This anxiety-provoking scenario leads other parents to a level of discomfort that makes providing social support very difficult for the nonbereaved parent and completely inadequate for the needs of the bereaved parent.

The griefwork of the bereaved parents involves numerous tasks:

... accept the reality of the loss, ventilate the emotions the grief raises, find new attachments by which to reorient their lives, find ways of reestablishing a sense of competence, integrate the loss into a philosophy of life, learn the pitfalls with the social role of a bereaved parent, rework the relationship

END-OF-LIFE CARE FOR CHILDREN WITH SPECIAL NEEDS AND THEIR FAMILIES

with the child's other parent, separate out their inner representations of
the child, and internalize the representation of the dead child. (Klass, 1988,
p. 152)

The bereaved parent, then, needs empathy and support from the caregiver
as he or she learns these new skills and constructs this new self. Caregivers
who have taken care of a dying child are not likely to be equipped to give all
of the support that these parents need, especially if the caregiver is a parent
who has never had a child die. An important intervention may be a referral to
a support group of other bereaved parents (see Resources section) or a referral
to a private therapist for help. It is important to remember the length of time
that grief lasts; Klass (described the initial phase of dramatic grief symptoms as
lasting somewhere around one year, and three years as a time frame for lesser
symptoms. However, he also stated that "parental bereavement is a permanent
condition" (p. 13), so that expectations that a parent will get over the death
and move on with life as before are not realistic ones for either the caregiver
or the bereaved parent to have. Such words as "closure" and "resolution" are
often used by the public – but not by bereaved parents.

A child's reaction to the death of a sibling must be examined in relationship to the child's concept of death and developmental status. This is far from
an uncommon occurrence, in that "approximately 1.8 million children from
birth to 18 years old are bereaved sibling in the United States at any given
time" (Hogan, 2008, p. 159). Interestingly, there is no English word for these
children, just as there is no term for their parents. These bereaved siblings
must cope with a host of issues, not least of which are distressing physical problems. Hogan described problems such as "headaches, stomachaches,
jumpiness or being clingy and fearful ... sleep difficulties ... attention deficit
and ... trouble concentrating ... they may feel lonely and isolated because no
one understands what they are going through ... hopelessness, anger, guilt,
fear and profound sadness" (p. 163).

Bereaved siblings who have lost a brother or sister with special needs must
do a risk assessment of their own health status. Are they at risk of dying from
whatever their sibling's cause of death was? Is the sibling's special need the
result of genetic influences that they may also carry, leading to speculation
about their ability to have healthy biological children someday? If the bereaved
sibling is the one with special needs, and a healthy sibling has died, what sense
can the bereaved child make of the brother or sister's death?

In addition to this risk assessment, bereaved siblings have lost the family they
previously had, because their parents are consumed with their own grief and
less available to them. "The home life of bereaved siblings is often enveloped
in a shroud of sadness"(Hogan, 2008, p. 164). Siblings have lost a brother or
sister, but they have also, in a sense, lost the parents they once had. Sibling

relationships are complicated, "typically fraught with conflicting feelings that ebb and flow" (Hogan, p. 164). Siblings can be close, or distant, and may take on roles within the family that, after a death, are difficult for the surviving siblings to fill themselves or to give up. A sibling may be a mentor or a tormentor, a hero or a worshipper, a good or bad example, a buffer between a sibling and the world, a protector or a bully, a fashion expert or the creator of hand-me-downs, a holder of secrets or a tattletale to parents. It is the ambivalence of the sibling relationship that leads to much of the bereaved sibling's regret and guilt.

As the bereaved parents think painfully about developmental milestones that the dead child will not meet, bereaved siblings are sadly aware of these milestones as well. The bereaved sibling is reminded of "the absence of the dead sibling at family reunions, births, marriages, graduations, and other rites of passage" (Hogan, 2008, p. 164). There are nearly constant reminders that the child is growing up, without the dead sibling's presence. If the bereaved sibling is very young when the brother or sister dies, the young survivor is likely not to understand the concepts of finality and universality, but those concepts, in a very personal manner, will become clear to the young child as he or she continues to develop. It is quite different to begin to develop a mature concept of death as an intellectual exercise, and entirely another to develop that mature concept because a sibling close to one's own age has died. Realizing more of what has been lost over time is a very painful developmental process.

Bereaved siblings will live with the death of their siblings longer than their parents will. At some point, siblings who lose an older brother or sister will eventually be older than their dead brother or sister ever became, which gives the survivor a peculiar sensation of usurping a family role to which he or she is not entitled.

Hogan (2008), while acknowledging that some surviving siblings get stuck in sadness and despair, also described positive meanings that bereaved siblings can find in their lives:

Resilient survivors develop an outlook on life that is optimistic. They are grateful for things that their peers take for granted. They have a renewed sense of being hopeful about the future. They sense that they have survived the worst and are better able to cope with difficult times. In essence, they believe that in coping with their sibling's death, they learned to trust their ability and inner strength to cope with future traumatic life events (p. 169).

Caregivers must be sensitive to the needs of the bereaved sibling. The child's developmental level, the level of understanding of the concept of death, and the relationship that the child had with the dead brother or sister are all important considerations as the survivor learns to cope with all of the losses that have occurred with the death. The caregiver must offer empathy and support to

END-OF-LIFE CARE FOR CHILDREN WITH SPECIAL NEEDS AND THEIR FAMILIES

the bereaved child, maintaining a sense of optimism that coping and finding meaning in life are possible. If a bereaved child is in school, caregivers should help families notify the child's school nurse and school counselor about the sibling's death. Because bereavement has physiological and cognitive effects, the school nurse needs to know that the child is bereaved so that he or she can help the child sort out the grief effects on the body and differentiate those effects from acute illness from other causes. Hogan (2008) also advocated for nurses and counselors to offer "a quiet place for the child to retreat to for a few moments if a grief reaction occurs" (p. 169). It is important, too, to "help bereaved siblings anticipate difficult times and have faith that their grief will soften and they will find relief from the thoughts, feelings, and images associated with the early, acute period of grief" (p. 169).

It is important to assess when a bereaved child or adolescent is in trouble with his or her grief and needs referral:

> ... if they are stuck in sadness and distressing feelings of blaming themselves and others; they continue to be angry at themselves, others, and the world; they express ongoing feelings of guilt; or they have unrelenting fears that preoccupy their emotional life. Children and adolescents should be referred for professional counseling if they express a lack of will to live, indicate a desire to harm themselves, or are preoccupied with the belief that they are responsible for their sibling's death. (Hogan, 2008, p. 170)

A child's special needs make careful assessment of signs of trouble particularly important. If a child has difficulty with communication, he or she may not be able to express feelings as easily, and issues of self-destructive thoughts may not be clear. Remembering that the child with special needs already lives with challenges above and beyond the healthy child's developmental issues is important as the bereavement will add weight to those difficulties and make life less easily managed. Cognitive deficits will be made worse because bereavement causes difficulty in focusing and concentrating (Hogan, 2008), so a child's teacher needs to be made aware of the bereavement in case he or she needs to spend extra time with the child working on refocusing attention as grief intrudes.

The issues that occur when a friend and peer dies are similar to those experienced by bereaved siblings, with some notable differences. In childhood, friendship fills a number of needs, including needs for "nurturance, intimacy, support, companionship, and affection ... status, power, self-esteem, achievement, identity, and approval" (Noppe & Noppe, 2008, p. 176). Friends are chosen voluntarily and are a source of mostly positive interactions. "Because friends tend to share many characteristics in common – such as cohort gender, social class, interests, and abilities – they are sources of self-definition and affirmation of self-worth" (Noppe & Noppe, p. 178). Given the importance of the friendship relationship in the lives of young children, then, the death of a friend causes severe disruption in the lives of peers. It differs from a sibling loss in that "family rivalries are not present and the child's role in the family is not left in an ambiguous state" (Noppe & Noppe, p. 180). Silverman (2000) asserted that a grieving friend receives only minimal support and guidance, and there are few rituals for a child to engage in to commemorate the death of a childhood friend. Noppe and Noppe stated that "American culture is impatient with adult grief; children are expected to recover even more quickly from the loss of a friend" (p. 180). The problems inherent in immature concepts of death are applicable here; does the child understand that death means irreversible change, and a non-functional body? Or does the child believe that the dead child will come back to play, or that the dead child is functioning on some limited level elsewhere? The young child is likely to turn to parents for "support, information, and comfort . . . However, with the best of intentions, adults may not offer much information; may provide euphemistic explanations . . . ; or may fail to recognize symptoms of grief in their child" (p. 180). Children who have a friend die need care and support, the chance to ask questions, and recognition of their grief. A very important intervention caregivers can provide is acknowledgement of the child's feelings, providing open communication and honest answers to the child's questions, and support as the child struggles with changes in his or her concept of universal death that includes peers of the child's age.

For adolescents, friendship changes with the transitions of puberty, transition to middle and high school, and cognitive and emotional changes in adolescence (Noppe & Noppe, 2008). "Interactions occur with same-sex friends, opposite-sex friends, and romantic partners (heterosexual and homosexual), and in the context of larger groups" (p. 181).

Compared with childhood friendships, the enhanced reciprocity, intimacy, and psychological basis (as opposed to activity basis) of the adolescent friendship make the death of a friend a major challenge for a teenager's coping abilities. Adolescent friendships are characterized by stability – adolescents believe they will be "friends forever" – and death disrupts their assumptive model of their future . . . Adding to the complexity are the shocking, tragic ways in which many adolescents die, which shake friends, families, schools and communities to the core. Even if the adolescent dies from an illness, people are shocked because of their assumptions about the power of medical cures and their belief that death occurs only in later years (Noppe & Noppe, pp. 182–183).

Caregivers of adolescents have an important role in helping the adolescent grieving the death of a friend. Because families are usually the recipients of social support, but friends often are not, Noppe and Noppe suggested that a way that "adults can help children and adolescents is to simply acknowledge the loss and validate their grief, without pressuring them to display emotions that

END-OF-LIFE CARE FOR CHILDREN WITH SPECIAL NEEDS AND THEIR FAMILIES

they may not feel or are not comfortable exhibiting" (p. 186). For adolescents, it is even more vital for the caregiver to be honest, open, and available while still respecting the adolescent's need to be with other peers and to have private time to think. The caregiver can help the adolescent role-play conversations with peers that will invite support from those peers. For adolescents with special needs who may have fewer friends than healthy adolescents do, or a smaller peer group, the caregiver may be a vital resource to support the adolescent's sadness at having a true friend die.

Noppe and Noppe (2008) pointed out that loss of a friend can have many effects:

> For children and adolescents who have lost a friend, the experience with death and grief is a part of who they are and what they will become. A part of their identities will be forged out of sadness and pain from the death of their friend. But the outcome can be a life-affirming road map for their future, an appreciation of their loved one, and a new definition of the meaning of friendship and its value to their existence (p. 187).

The caregiver of a child with special needs has multiple roles in caring and supporting the family and surviving children after a death. Understanding how the child's concept of death develops is key to anticipating a bereaved child's questions, and understanding what happens to parents, bereaved siblings, and bereaved peers is crucial in anticipating their physiological, cognitive, emotional, social, and spiritual needs after a death. The caregiver must care for him- or herself first, so that he or she has the emotional strength and resources to support the family and child during their grief. Although there is much pain and sadness to cope with, there is also great resilience and courage to be found in a child's death and the family's ability to find a new life that does not forget the dead child, but holds fond memories and a new appreciation of the fragility and preciousness of life.

RESOURCES

There are a number of excellent books for bereaved parents and books to teach a child about death and to provide hope after the death of a loved person in a child's life. An abbreviated list follows:

For parents

Bernstein, J.R. (1998). *When the bough breaks: Forever after the death of a son or daughter*. Riverside, NJ: Andrews McMeel Publishing Company.
Mitchell, E. (2009). *Beyond tears: Living after losing a child* (rev. edition). New York: St. Martin's Griffin.

Redfern, S., & Gilbert, S.K. (2008). *The grieving garden: Living with the death of a child*. Newburyport, MA: Hampton Roads.

Rosof, B.D. (1995). *The worst loss: How families heal from the death of a child*. New York: Holt Paperbacks.

Schiff, H.S. (1978). The bereaved parent. New York: Penguin Books.

For children

Bunting, E. (1999). *Rudi's pond*. New York, NY: Clarion.

Buscaglia, L. (1982). *The fall of Freddie the leaf: A story of life for all ages*. Thorofare, NJ: Slack.

Ferguson, D. (1992). *A bunch of balloons*. Omaha, NE: Centering.

Grollman, E., & Johnson, J. (2006). *A complete book about death for kids*. Omaha, NE: Centering.

Gryte, M. (1988). *No new baby: For siblings who have a brother or sister die before birth* (Spanish version: *no tenremos un nuevo bebé*). Omaha, NE: Centering.

Heegard, M.E. (1988). *When someone very special dies*. Minneapolis, MN: Woodland Press.

Krasny Brown, L., & Brown, M. (1998). *When dinosaurs die: A guide to understanding death*. Boston: Little, Brown Books for Young Readers.

Muñoz-Kiehne, M. (2000). *Since my brother died* (Spanish version: *Desde que murió mi hermano*. Omaha, NE: Centering Corporation.

Old, W. (1995). *Stacy had a baby sister*. Morton Grove, IL: Albert Whitman.

Simon, J. (2001). *This book is for all kids, but especially my sister Libby. Libby died*. Austin, TX: Idea University Press.

Smith, H.I., & Johnson, J. (2006). *What does that mean? A dictionary of death, dying and grief terms for grieving children*. Omaha, NE: Centering.

Thomas, P. (2001). *I miss you: A first look at death*. Hauppauge, NY: Barron's Educational Series.

White, E.B. (1952). Charlotte's web. New York, NY: Harper.

There are also a number of web sites that offer help to caregivers, bereaved parents, and children.

For caregivers

American Hospice Foundation at www.americanhospice.org
Association for Death Education and Counseling at www.adec.org
Children's Hospice International at www.chionline.org
Hospice Foundation of America at www.hospicefoundation.org
The Initiative for Pediatric Palliative Care at www.ippcweb.org
National Hospice and Palliative Care Organization at www.nhpco.org

For parents

American Childhood Cancer Organization at www.acco.org/
Bereaved Parents of the USA at www.bereavedparentsusa.org

The Compassionate Friends at www.compassionatefriends.org
The MISS Foundation at www.missfoundation.org
Partnership for Parents at www.partnershipforparents.org

For children and adolescents

The Dougy Center at www.dougy.org
Growth House at www.growthhouse.org
KidsAid at www.kidsaid.com
National Alliance for Grieving Children at www.nationalallianceforgrievingchildren.org
SuperSibs! at www.supersibs.org
WillMar Center for Bereaved Children at www.willmarcenter.org

REFERENCES

American Heart Association. (2005). International Consensus Conference on Cardiopulmonary Resuscitation and Emergency Cardiovascular Care Science with Treatment Recommendations. *Circulation, 112*: III5–III16.

Balk, D. (2008). The adolescent's encounter with death. In K.J. Doka & A.S. Tucci (Eds.), *Living with grief: Children and adolescents* (pp. 25–42). Washington, DC: Hospice Foundation of America.

Beale, E.A., Baile, W.F., & Aaron, J. (2005). Silence is not golden: Communicating with children dying from cancer. *Journal of Clinical Oncology, 23*(15), 3629–3631.

Bluebond-Langner, M. (1978). *The private worlds of dying children*. Princeton, NJ: Princeton University Press.

Cassileth, B.R., Zupkis, R.V., Sutton-Smith, K., & March, V. (1980). Information and participation preferences among cancer patients. *Annals of Internal Medicine, 92*, 832–836.

Centers for Disease Control. (2010). National Center for Health Statistics. Retrieved from http://www.cdc.gov/nchs/deaths.htm.

Corr, C.A. (1996). Children, development and encounters with death and bereavement. In C.A. Corr & D.M. Corr (Eds.), *Handbook of childhood death and bereavement* (pp. 3–28). New York, NY: Springer.

Corr, C.A. (2008). Children's emerging awareness of death. In K.J. Doka & A.S. Tucci (Eds.), *Living with grief: Children and adolescents* (pp. 5–17). Washington, DC: Hospice Foundation of America.

Davies, B., Cook, K., O'Loane, M., et al. (1996). Caring for dying children: Nurses' experiences. *Pediatric Nursing, 22*(6), 500–507.

Doka, K.J. (1982). The social organization of terminal care in the pediatric hospitals. *Omega, 12*, 345–354.

Doka, K.J. (1996). The cruel paradox: Children who are living with life-threatening illnesses. In C.A. Corr & D.M. Corr (Eds.), *Handbook of childhood death and bereavement* (pp. 89–105). New York, NY: Springer.

Dunsmore, J., & Quine, S. (1995). Information, support, and decision-making needs and preferences of adolescents with cancer: Implications for health professionals. *Journal of Psychosocial Oncology, 13*(4), 39–56.

Grollman, E.A. (1995). Grieving children: Can we answer their questions? In K.J. Doka (Ed.), *Children mourning, mourning children* (pp. 17–27). Washington, DC: Hospice Foundation of America.

Gunther, J. (1949). *Death be not proud: A memoir.* New York, NY: Harper & Row.

Hogan, N. (2008). Sibling loss: Issues for children and adolescents. In K.J. Doka & A.S. Tucci (Eds.), *Living with grief: Children and adolescents* (pp. 159–174). Washington, DC: Hospice Foundation.

Kane, B. (1979). Children's concepts of death. *Journal of Genetic Psychology, 134,* 141–153.

Keene, E.A., Hutton, N., Hall, B., & Rushton, C. Bereavement debriefing sessions: An intervention to support health professionals in managing their grief after the death of a patient. *Pediatric Nursing, 36*(4), 185–189.

Klass, D. (1988). *Parental grief: Solace and resolution.* New York, NY: Springer.

Noppe, I.C., & Noppe, L.D. (2008). When a friend dies. In K.J. Doka & A.S. Tucci (Eds.), *Living with grief: Children and adolescents* (pp. 175–192). Washington, DC: Hospice Foundation of America.

Noppe, L.D., & Noppe, I.C. (1996). Ambiguity in adolescent understandings of death. In C.A. Corr & D.E. Balk (Eds.), *Handbook of adolescent death and bereavement* (pp. 25–41). New York, NY: Springer.

Papadatou, D. (2000). A proposed model of health professionals' grieving process. *Omega, 41*(1), 59–77.

Piaget, J. (1929). *The child's conception of the world.* London, UK: Routledge & Kegan Paul.

Silverman, P.R. (2000). *Never too young to know: Death in children's lives.* New York, NY: Oxford University Press.

Speece, M.W., & Brent, S.B. (1996). The development of children's understanding of death. In C.A. Corr & D.M Corr (Eds.), *Handbook of childhood death and bereavement* (pp. 29–50). New York, NY: Springer.

Stevens, M.M., & Dunsmore, J.C. (1996). Adolescents who are living with a life-threatening illness. In C.A. Corr & D.E. Balk (Eds.), *Handbook of adolescent death and bereavement* (pp. 107–135). New York, NY: Springer.

END-OF-LIFE CARE FOR CHILDREN
WITH SPECIAL NEEDS AND THEIR
FAMILIES

CHAPTER 13

ASSESSMENT, AND DEVELOPMENT OF AN INTERPROFESSIONAL PLAN OF CARE

Nancy Lowry and Patricia Shaw

Caring for Children with Special Healthcare Needs and Their Families: A Handbook for Healthcare Professionals, First Edition. Edited by Linda L. Eddy.
© 2013 John Wiley & Sons, Inc. Published 2013 by John Wiley & Sons, Inc.

Nurses and other healthcare professionals who have the privilege of working with children and youth with special health needs (CYSHN) and their families are in a unique position to assure coordination of care among providers. A well-thought out plan of care is a key to the collaborative, interdisciplinary process that is essential to meeting the child's needs appropriately.

The foundation for developing the care plan for a child with special health needs begins with a thorough documentation of the child's health history, followed by a comprehensive assessment (Burns & Kodadek, 2009). It is critical to understand how the activities of surveillance, screening and assessment fit into this process (Lipkin, 2011).

Surveillance is the process of recognizing children who may be at risk of developmental delays or health conditions (Lipkin,2011). Surveillance includes taking a health history from a parent, and observing the child's development. The purpose of surveillance is to identify children who may have a condition, and need to have a specific screening or assessment done. For example, a school nurse reviews all immunization records in his or her assigned schools to identify children who have not received all of the necessary immunizations. The nurse would then contact parents to notify them of the need to update their child's immunizations.

Screening involves using a standardized tool with recognized reliability, validity, sensitivity, and specificity to identify children who have a high likelihood of having a health or developmental condition. Surveillance may occur at every contact with a child, whereas screening occurs at periodic intervals. An example of screening would be the administration of the Ages and Stages (ASQ) developmental screen at specific intervals on all babies in the nurse's caseload who were born prematurely. Any babies with abnormal screen results would be referred for a developmental assessment.

Assessment is a comprehensive process aimed at identifying specific health or developmental disorders (Lipkin, 2011). Assessment may include a head-to-toe physical examination, as well as the use of focused assessments such as evaluation of feeding and nutritional status in a child with cerebral palsy. Surveillance and screening can be performed by a variety of providers such as an early intervention provider, audiologist, or nurse. Assessment is a more comprehensive process that should be completed by a professional with the education and professional scope of practice that is specific to the area of assessment.

Exemplar: The identification of newborns with a potential hearing loss illustrates the use of all three of the above processes. In many states, hospitals are mandated to conduct **surveillance** by testing all newborns with a standardized device that checks for otoacoustic emissions (OAE). These screenings may be performed by a nursing assistant, volunteer, or sometimes by a nurse. If the baby passes the screen in both ears, the parents are given the results. If a baby fails the screen in one or more ears, the parents are referred to a provider in their community who does a second level of hearing **screening** with a different test, often the automated brain response (ABR). If the baby fails the second level of testing, the parents are then referred to a pediatric audiologist who conducts a comprehensive **assessment** of the baby's hearing loss and need for amplification. A care coordinator can be very helpful to the family during this process by explaining the different levels of testing and removing barriers to needed follow-up such as transportation and insurance coverage (Smith & Bazini, 2003). The coordinator would also refer the baby to early intervention and parent support providers such as the national "Guide By Your Side" organization that provides trained parent mentors who also have a hearing impaired child.

THE ASSESSMENT PROCESS

Assessment is not a single activity. It is a process, which begins with family engagement and ultimately results in a comprehensive plan of care on which the provider and family can agree. Once the plan of care is implemented, the provider will be continually assessing its effectiveness and planning additional interventions. A comprehensive assessment of a child and family with complex needs may require more than one visit to complete. It is important to consider the child in the context of his or her environment when conducting an assessment. The advantage of this holistic approach is the identification of social or cultural needs that have potential to influence the care a family provides for the child.

Preparing for your visit with the family

The assessment process begins before your actual meeting with the parents and child. Review the referral information that you have received. Review any medical or school records that have been received to identify whether specific screenings or assessments have already been completed. Depending on your role, you may have received very basic and incomplete information on an unplanned emergency admission to an acute care unit. Your first priority will be to assess the child for urgent physical needs and begin to implement the physician's orders. In a setting such as a public health department or primary care office, you will usually have more time to prepare for your first meeting

ASSESSMENT, AND DEVELOPMENT
OF AN INTERPROFESSIONAL PLAN
OF CARE

with family. If the child has a diagnosis with which you are not familiar, such as a rare genetic condition, it is vital that you do some minimal research on the condition so that you can gather appropriate information during your assessment. Table 13.1 lists some credible sources for information. When a child has a rare condition, parents know that they will constantly have to explain their child's diagnosis. You will gain a great deal of respect and credibility from the parents if you have taken the time to research the condition. It is also important to research the most current treatment and long-term prognosis for conditions that you may have heard of, such as Down syndrome or autism, because the care and prognosis for many conditions have changed dramatically. Taking a moment to consider what it might be like to be that child or parent is also important, and helps assure a thoughtful and empathetic approach.

Practice tips: Finding reliable information on the Internet

- **A useful tool** for determining whether a health-related web site is credible is the Trust It or Trash It web site that was developed by the Genetic Alliance. http://www.trustortrash.org/TrustorTrash.pdf

- **Look for an "About Us" section** to see who owns the site. Commercial sites often have their own interests such as selling a particular product, and this may influence the accuracy of the information presented. Web addresses ending in ".org," ".edu," or ".gov" are more likely to contain unbiased information (CaCoon Health Notes, 2011; Genetic Alliance, 2012).

- **Be a skeptic.** If it seems too good to be true, it is probably not true.

- **Look for credible research.** Look for evidence that the authors have clinical experience with the condition and for whether their work has been replicated by other research.

- **Make sure the information is current.** Look to see when the web site was most recently updated.

- **You can "Google" the name of a condition by** using the phases for "health care guidelines for CONDITION NAME" or "critical elements of care for CONDITION NAME." These phrases are more likely to turn up credible information than simply searching for the name of the condition alone.

- **Find a medical library.** Some medical libraries are accessible to the public. To find medical libraries in your area go to www.nnlm.gov/members/adv.html.

ASSESSMENT, AND DEVELOPMENT OF AN INTERPROFESSIONAL PLAN OF CARE

Search by geographic location, and select "Only institutions that serve health care consumers."

- See Table 13.1 for a list of reliable websites.

Table 13.1 Reliable Web Sites for Researching Health Conditions

American Academy of Pediatrics	www.aap.org
EthnoMed	www.ethnomed.org
Genetic Alliance	www.geneticalliance.org
MedlinePlus	www.medlineplus.gov
National Guideline Clearinghouse	www.guideline.gov
National Organization for Rare Disorders (NORD)	www.rarediseases.org
New York Online Access to Health	www.noah-health.org
PubMed	www.pubmed.gov

Cultural considerations and the use of interpreters

It is important to know something about the family's cultural background. All families have their own "culture." Some bring a broader cultural perspective based on their country of origin, heritage, or socioeconomic status. For example, a family may have religious and cultural beliefs that support using other medical approaches instead of accessing traditional American/Western medicine, and may believe that prayer alone will cure their child's cancer. In addition, many recent immigrants to the United States come from countries where medical care, other than emergent care, was not available, and decisions about which treatments to pursue may have been made by a medical provider, healer, or other authority figure. Families arrive in the United States only to be confronted by a seemingly unlimited number of choices regarding treatment for a specific condition. They do not have the knowledge or cultural experience that prepares them to make these choices, and so they may acquiesce to the physician or a senior respected member of their community.

You should always ask if a family requires an interpreter to communicate. As a requirement of Title VI of the Civil Rights Act of 1964, interpreter services are to be provided to limited-English-proficient patients at no cost to the patient. All recipients of federal funds must comply with this requirement (Hoffman, 2011).

Language barriers and the use of interpreters can affect the communication and understanding of information that is shared as well as the client/family-nurse relationship. Utilizing professional medical interpreter services whenever possible enhances the potential for information being relayed and received accurately by both the parent and the provider. Interpreters often are helpful resources for the provider, as they can explain cultural nuances, and share knowledge of resources in the family's cultural community.

Practice Tip: The following tips can be useful when working with an interpreter:(Lipson & Dibble, 2005; CaCoon Program Manual, 2012)

- Ascertain whether the person will need an interpreter. This information is often available on the referral. In some countries, several different dialects are spoken, and it may take extra time to arrange for an interpreter who speaks the correct dialect. Often, people who have lived in the United States for a while may have enough of a command of English for a simple interview to be conducted. They may tell you that they do not need an interpreter, but you should still use one if you are going to be discussing complex issues or obtaining consent for a medical procedure. Do not assume that people can read in English or in their primary language because they can speak the language. You should always inquire about their reading ability.

- Avoid use of children and family members as interpreters. Family members or children do not have the technical skills and language competence for medical interpretation. Family members may be biased, and having them interpret could violate the patient's confidentiality rights.

- Schedule adequate time for the visit. An interpreted appointment may take more than twice as long as an ordinary visit because accurate nterpretation often requires long explanatory phrases.

- Whenever possible, meet with the interpreter before the session to explain the purpose of your visit. If the interpreter knows the topics that you will be discussing, it gives the interpreter time to consider how he or she might convey the information. Interpreters can also often explain the belief systems and cultural nuances that a person from a particular culture may have.

- Avoid technical terminology, abbreviations, jargon, slang, and metaphors.

- Look at and speak directly to the person, not the interpreter. Ask the person, "what do you think about this plan", rather than asking the interpreter to ask the person what they think about the plan.

- Interpreters will only interpret what the provider and the person say. Encourage the interpreter to refrain from inserting his or her own ideas or interpretations, or omitting information.

ASSESSMENT, AND DEVELOPMENT OF AN INTERPROFESSIONAL PLAN OF CARE

- Check the person's understanding by asking the person to repeat the message or instructions in his or her own words.

- Do not conduct side conversations when working with an interpreter. Interpreters, especially sign language interpreters, will interpret every word that is spoken during the meeting.

Family engagement – Getting to know the family and child

CYSHN and their families come into contact with nurses and other healthcare providers in a variety of settings that include hospitals, primary care clinics, early intervention centers, specialty care clinics, WIC, schools, and the home.

How the nurse introduces his- or herself and the role the nurse will have while working with the family is crucial. When explaining services being offered, it is imperative that the provider convey to the family that the potential relationship is a shared partnership. The providers' role is one of empowerment, supporting the family in developing their role as advocates for their child. The tone used by the nurse/provider can enhance or discourage a positive working relationship with a family.

One of the keys to successful engagement with a family is to respond quickly when they are referred for services. "[I]t can be very painful for parents to discover that their child has special needs when they did not expect it... it is important that parents receive emotional support when they first learn of their child's condition" (Narramore, 2008). It is ideal for the nurse or care coordinator to be introduced to the family as soon as possible after a diagnosis is made, or even prior, when testing is being done. Including the care coordinator in case staffing and discharge planning will help assure a smooth transition when it is time for discharge. An example is a preterm infant admitted to the NICU. There is often much unknown for weeks about what the future holds for the infant.

The NICU environment can be intimidating, and there may be many ups and downs related to the child's condition. Many of the referrals for services for CYSHN come from hospital NICUS.

It is ideal if the care coordinator for services after discharge be identified early in the hospitalization. Including the public health nurse or other community provider in discharge planning will help assure a smooth transition to home for the child and family. Parents of premature infants often have immediate needs for assistance with transportation, childcare for older siblings, pet care, food, and other basic needs. The unexpected/untimely nature of a premature delivery is very much a crisis for families on many levels, both practical and emotional.

Decision-making processes are often impaired due to enormous stress and grief. Having a consistent coordinator of care who can interpret medical information, help with scheduling of follow-up appointments, etc., and provide emotional support can help families cope as they navigate the challenges of parenting a special needs child.

Developing a therapeutic relationship with a family is often challenging but also rewarding. When home visiting services are offered, parents often feel vulnerable and must make a decision that is based on their assessment of the risk of allowing a professional to enter their life and a comparison of the perceived risks to the benefit that they may gain from the relationship (Jack, DiCenso, & Lohfeld, 2005). Families often engage in a process to limit their vulnerability through a three-stage process that includes overcoming their fear, developing trust, and seeking mutuality. The parent may make a special effort to clean their house and make sure the baby is dressed in his or her best clothes; they may ask other family members or a friend to be present during the visit. Trust is established once the parent feels that they will not be judged and that the nurse or home visitor is willing to work on shared goals that include the parent's perspective.

Mutuality can be promoted by having the home visitor share parts of his or her life. Parents will often ask if the visitor has children as this allows them to gauge whether the visitor understands the challenges of raising children. The speed at which families and professionals move through the phases depends on the interpersonal skills and experiences of both the visitor and the parents. Visitors who are able to project an attitude of acceptance and openness will be most successful in establishing a therapeutic relationship. Some families will be able to develop trust by the end of the first or second visit; other parents who have experienced many disrupted relationships in their lives may allow the professional to continue visiting but will never develop a trusting relationship.

Practice Tip: Strategies to facilitate an effective relationship with families

- Use an interpreter if needed.

- Welcome anyone who the parent has invited to attend the visit.

- Providers need to be knowledgeable about the challenges faced by children with special needs, as well as having up-to-date information on the child's specific condition. Parents appreciate it when a provider has taken the time to learn about their child. Giving a family practical information about their child's condition, or directing them to helpful resources helps to build trust in the provider.

- Flexibility and an ability to accept families who may have a different standard of household organization or cleanliness, or a different value system, will also aid in relationship building.

- Listen to families and engage them in developing a shared plan of care. You are working *with* the parent, not delivering a service *to* the family. Healthcare providers often discount a parent's observations about a child, but parents know their child best and often notice subtle signs of a change in their child's health that are not always apparent during an office visit. Ask parents why they do their child's care in a different way than the way they were taught in the hospital. The parents may have developed a method that works well for them, or they may have had to modify the procedure because they do not have the necessary resources to purchase supplies or equipment.

- Develop a clear sense of boundaries in relationships with families. Your role is to teach the families how to advocate for their needs, not create dependency on the home visitor to meet all of the family's needs.

The assessment process

You should always begin your initial visit by introducing yourself. Explain your role, and explain which agency you work for. Tell the family the purpose of your visit. Briefly explain what you would like to accomplish during the visit. At this point, you need to ask the family what their goals are for the visit and ask if they have any questions. When you begin to gather the history from the parent, review what you already know from the referral so that parents do not have to repeat their whole story. Observe the child while you are completing the health history with the parents. You can observe a lot about the child – the child's general state of health, his or her awareness, and ability to interact with the environment. Is the child awake or sleeping? Is the child able to interact verbally or nonverbally with other people in the room? What is the child's position, muscle tone, and gait? What methods does the child use to communicate with family members? If you are doing a home visit, use all of your senses while conducting your visit. Take note of the neighborhood, type and condition of housing, and possible safety hazards. Notice how people are dressed. Note the condition of the apartment or house – is it cluttered or organized? Is there a strong smell of tobacco? Are there pets in the home? Is the family expecting you and ready for your visit, or are they hesitant and unsure whether they want you to be there?

A comprehensive assessment includes taking a complete health and developmental history, as well as performing a physical assessment and focused assessments such as on nutrition and feeding. The scope of the assessment process is dependent upon the provider's experience, education, licensure, and scope of practice.

Components of the health history (Burns & Kodadek, 2009) include the following:

- Patient-identifying information

- History of current illness

- Past medical history – prenatal and postnatal, past illnesses and injuries, allergies, hospitalizations and emergency room visits, nutrition, growth, development, nutrition history, and current medications

- Review of symptoms

- Family history

- Socioeconomic – housing, employment, health insurance coverage, general relationship between family members, extended family supports, use of other community agencies

It is important to use screening and assessment tools that are standardized. The resource section at the end of this chapter outlines several suggested tools that are appropriate for use with CSHCN. If you are screening a child to determine if a referral to early intervention is needed, it is a good idea to find out which screening instruments the early intervention program accepts as evidence of a potential delay.

Common issues in children with special needs

Medical complexity. Children with special needs often have multiple conditions. According to the 2005/2006 National Survey of Children with Special Health Care Needs (CAHMI, 2012), 91% of CSHCN have one or more conditions on a list of 16 common conditions, and 25% of CSHCN have three or more of these conditions. For example a child with athetoid cerebral palsy may have motor delays, as well as nutritional and elimination disorders. This child may also have a seizure disorder and associated dental problems that are related to the long-term use of anticonvulsants.

In addition, many children are technology-dependent and require the use of ventilators, nebulizers, feeding tubes, or dialysis at home. This medical complexity places additional emotional, physical, financial, and environmental strains on the parents and siblings, which may dramatically alter the family's previous lifestyle. Families may need to move to a different house or neighborhood. They may decide to move from a rural to an urban area to be closer to care. If they decide to continue living in a remote area, steps must be taken to obtain a backup generator if the child is technology-dependent. Families living in remote areas may not have access to in-home nursing care, which causes increased exhaustion for family members who must provide continuous care. One helpful intervention is to assist the family to contact their utility and phone providers about their child's need for technology at home. When utility companies are provided with medical documentation, they can indicate by placing a sticker on the house meter that a family's power is not to be turned off for nonpayment of a bill. The utility company will work on a payment plan with the family. In the event of a power outage, when feasible, the power company may be able to prioritize emergency repairs to a neighborhood where a technology-dependent person is living. The emergency plan for a child needs to include what the backup plan for emergencies will be. Does the family have a backup power source? Will the child need to be moved to another family member's house or readmitted to the hospital until the power is restored?

Other stressors on a family who is caring for a child with multiple conditions is that the family must deal with attending multiple clinics with multiple providers, who sometimes seem to offer conflicting advice. The family may need to travel to a distant city to attend a specialty clinic so that transportation, lodging and insurance coverage may become barriers to receiving care.

Developmental and intellectual disabilities. It is estimated that 12–13% of children have a developmental or behavioral disorder, whereas intellectual disabilities may affect as many as one child in 83 (Lipkin, 2011). These children will need early intervention, special education, and long-term occupational, physical, or speech therapies. The nurse or other provider who is working with young children should be skilled at performing developmental screenings and assessments. Some examples of standardized screening and assessment tools include the following:

- Ages and Stages Questionnaire

- Ages and Stages Social/Emotional Paul H. Brookes Publishing Co. (800) 638–3775; www.pbrookes.com

- Bayley Infant Neurodevelopmental screeneer (BINS) http://www.pearson assessments.com

- Modified Checklist for Autism in Toddlers (M-CHAT) http://www2.gsu. edu/~psydlr/DianaLRobins/Official_M- CHAT_Website_files/M-CHAT.pdf

ASSESSMENT, AND DEVELOPMENT OF AN INTERPROFESSIONAL PLAN OF CARE

Alterations in nutritional status. Nutrition concerns in CYSHN are encountered frequently, and these nutrition disorders are likely to become chronic over time. Common concerns include:

- Alterations in growth – underweight, overweight, or short stature

- Inadequate energy and nutrient intake to support growth and health

- Feeding problems related to oral-motor and/or behavioral difficulties

- Medication-nutrient interactions and need for enteral tube feedings (Lucas, Feucht, & Geiger, 2004)

A standardized screening tool should be utilized to elicit the parents' concerns about nutrition. Growth should be plotted at regular intervals on a standardized growth chart. The nurse should know where to refer children for a comprehensive nutritional assessment and feeding therapy if indicated. In some rural communities, It can be difficult to locate a nutritionist who has expertise in CSHCN. The local WIC nutritionist or the closest pediatric hospital may be able to direct you to an appropriate provider.

The following resources will be helpful in determining which growth grid is most appropriate for a child:

- "A Look at Diet and Health" Nutrition Screening for CSHCN – see tool in this chapter, or at the following Web site: Regional and Statewide Services for Students with orthopedic Impairments http://www.rsoi.org/Pages/SampleFeedingForms.aspx

- CDC growth charts http://www.cdc.gov/growthcharts/

- Washington State Department of Health Nutrition Interventions for Children with Special Needs (2010) http://here.doh.wa.gov/materials/nutrition-interventions

- Nutrition for children with special health care needs; A self study curriculum http://depts.washington.edu/pwdlearn/web/

- Down syndrome growth charts http://www.growthcharts.com/charts/DS/charts.htm

Pain. Pain in CSHCN may be under-recognized because of the child's inability to communicate or because a provider does not understand how a child's particular disability may contribute to pain. Children with sickle cell disease or juvenile rheumatoid arthritis are easily recognized. Children with cerebral palsy may have less-obvious pain caused by dislocated hips, joint contractures,

GERD, or an improperly fitted wheelchair or orthotics. The provider can learn more about pediatric pain management and appropriate screening tools at this Web site:

The Centre for Pediatric Pain Research in the IWK Health Centre, in Halifax, Nova Scotia, Canada at Dalhousie University. http://pediatric-pain.ca/

Sleep. Sleep problems are commonly encountered in CSHCN. Presenting concerns often include difficulty falling and/or staying asleep, irregular sleep-wake patterns, early morning awakenings, and poor sleep routines. Pain, nutritional concerns, and neurological disorders can also contribute to disruptions in sleep patterns. Sleep disorders are often very difficult for parents to manage and result in increased exhaustion for parents and siblings as well.

Behavioral concerns. Children may have a diagnosis of attention deficit hyperactivity disorder (ADHD), bipolar disorder, or oppositional defiant disorder as a primary diagnosis. Other children with specific genetic syndromes may exhibit behavioral symptoms as well. Issues with limited access to care and a shortage of mental health providers who understand the complexities of mental health issues in children who also have chronic physical or developmental disorders cause difficult access to care for many families. Insurance coverage for behavioral health is often limited. The American Academy of Pediatrics Bright Futures Web site has helpful information on screening for behavioral disorders: http://brightfutures.aap.org/.

Family assessment. A comprehensive assessment must include an evaluation of families' strengths, priorities, and needs. If the provider approaches the family from the perspective that the parents are the expert about their child and that the parents and provider are entering into a shared partnership, the family is much more likely to engage in an ongoing relationship with the provider (Young, 1998). Discussing roles and relationships is often difficult for parents who not know the provider well, so it is better to start with assessing child health issues first. There are several checklists and tools that can assist the provider in understanding family needs, such as the Family Needs Survey, which has been adapted from Carl Dunst. It is available at the Advancing Milestones Web site: http://www.advancingmilestones.com/PDFs/m_resources_family-needs-survey.pdf.

An effective tool that can be used to determine the complexity of a child's and family's needs is known as the Tier Tool. This tool measures the acuity of needs in 13 domains. A score is given in each domain. The domain scores are then added to arrive at a tier level of 1, 2, or 3. This tool can be used to develop the plan of care and prioritize interventions with families. The tier tool can assist the provider and family in agreeing on a list of areas that need to be addressed (a problem list) and deciding on which areas are priorities to be addressed first. A link to this tool is included in the resource section at the end of this chapter.

DEVELOPING A PLAN OF CARE

Once the assessment is completed, the provider needs to synthesize the information and develop a plan of care that will meet the child's and family's goals. Interventions should be evidence-based when possible. Interventions may also be based on the provider's clinical experience and judgment based on years of experience, knowledge of resources available in the community where the family resides, and knowledge of cultural practices.

Including the parents and the CYSHCN (if the child's age and condition allows) when developing the plan of care is crucial. It is important for the provider to keep in mind that parents experience grief when they learn of their child's condition, and their grief can recur intermittently throughout the trajectory of their child's life. The stage of grief the parents are in can impact their ability to contribute to the care-planning process (Narramore, 2008). Family support, respite, and counseling should all be considered for inclusion in the plan of care, with one primary goal being to decrease the social isolation that is so common with parents of CYSHCN.

Key components of a care plan

A care plan is intended to be a guide to providers of many disciplines who are working with CYSHCN. In the hospital setting, an up-to-date care plan is essential for communicating between providers in order to assure continuity of care across all shifts. At a glance, a provider can see the date/time when an entry was made, helping to understand the current status of the child, what issues have been resolved, and what continues to need monitoring or attention. A care plan should include at the very minimum:

- A brief statement for each problem (example: poor nutrition status)

- Planned interventions and who will be responsible for each intervention

- Expected and actual outcomes for each intervention

Role of the care coordinator in developing and carrying out the plan of care

The influence a nurse care coordinator on the formation of the plan of care cannot be emphasized enough. This role will vary between settings – hospital versus community – as will the degree the family is involved in the decisions around the plan for care. The nurse, using keen assessment skills, can ascertain the family's needs, assuring they are considered whenever possible, especially at the time of discharge for hospitalized children. He or she can assist the family by interpreting medical information; assessing the family's practical needs; and connecting the family to resources such as transportation, financial assistance, and respite care. Perhaps of most importance is the emotional support offered to a family at a critical time, as well as referring the parents for ongoing support.

Ideally the care plan will be interdisciplinary – with multiple providers giving input, updating the plan, and reviewing the entries other disciplines have made. For example, a preemie may have entries made to his/her care plan by the physician, clinical nurse specialist, bedside nurse; dietician, physical or occupational therapists, and medical specialists. Working from the same care plan is easier in a hospital setting where providers are documenting in the same chart or electronic record. Once the child is home and receiving ambulatory and community-based services, it is challenging for providers to share the same care plan.

Once the provider and the family have arrived at an agreed-upon set of interventions, the provider must determine which interventions should occur first. It is helpful to prioritize according to the urgency of the situation. The highest priority should be given to issues that impact the basic health and safety of the child. If a child is acutely ill, the child must receive urgent medical care. The next priority should be to assure that the family's basic needs are being met because without basic resources, a family will not be able to focus on other areas. Basic needs include resources such as adequate housing, food, transportation, and utilities.

Once these resources are in place, the child's needs for primary care and specialty care, and health insurance can be addressed. Finally, referrals to community agencies such as early intervention, special education, and mental health services can be addressed with the family.

Example of a problem and possible interventions

Problem statement: child has not received the recommended well-child care because the family lacks transportation. The provider's care plan might include the following interventions:

By October 31, 2011

ASSESSMENT, AND DEVELOPMENT
OF AN INTERPROFESSIONAL PLAN
OF CARE

Goals

1. Identify urgent unmet medical needs

2. Identify family barriers to meeting needs

3. Develop plan with family to overcome one barrier

4. Evaluate/monitor the plan with family

Interventions:

- Linked mom to primary care provider for well-child care, made call for her, scheduled appointment, modeled for mom client scheduling. Receptionist said if family was "no show" the provider would not see them again.

- Reinforced with mom need to keep appointments or cancel the day before.

- Mom says that schedules are hard to keep for her. Developed large calendar with PCP appointment, contact number

- Demonstrated scheduling Dial a Ride with mom and arranged for transport to next appointment, modeling how to schedule ride/left number on calendar.

- Scheduled next HV for 2 days before PCP visit to monitor plan.

Documentation and the use of electronic health records

The provider's assessment, plan of care, interventions, and outcomes must be documented in the child's record in a concise and logical order. The documentation must meet the legal requirements for health records, whether the record is a paper chart or part of an electronic health record (EHR). The purposes for a health record include the following (Austin, 2006):

- It provides a method for communication among multiple providers in a health system or community agency who may be caring for a child

- It can be used to facilitate and substantiate the billing process

- It may be used to provide data for research purposes

- It should be organized in a manner that will facilitate chart audits, or other quality assurance activities

- It is a legal document that can be used to provide evidence for disability determinations, malpractice lawsuits, and workers compensation

ASSESSMENT, AND DEVELOPMENT OF AN INTERPROFESSIONAL PLAN OF CARE

Practice tip: What to include in the EHR

In order to achieve the preceding goals, the record should contain the following minimum requirements:

- Patient identification including full name, birthdate, address, and contact information; next of kin; and names of decision makers for care provided (in the case of a child, this would be the child's parents, guardians, or other people who have the legal right to make healthcare decisions)

- Many community agencies also include a family database, which outlines the family composition, as well as a list of family strengths and needs

- A problem list including past and current medical and nursing diagnoses with the date indicated for initial diagnosis and the date the problem was resolved

- Narrative notes or checklists that outline the provider's nursing assessment, interventions, and contacts with families and other providers

- A care plan;

- Screening forms should be included in the chart. The forms must have the child's name, birthdate, and the date the screening was completed. The form should be completely filled out, signed, and dated by the provider who did the screening. The screening should have the score recorded, if the screening is one that is scored.

- In the case of paper records, seem agencies put together blank charts with all of the usual paperwork that is needed. Sometimes, a particular form will not be needed because it is not applicable for the age of the child or the child's condition. These blank forms should be removed from the chart – otherwise it may appear to a chart auditor that a provider left work undone that should have been completed.

- Releases of information and consents for treatment need to be in the record. If an interpreter was used during a visit, the fact that an interpreter was used should be included. It is especially important to note that an interpreter was used during the informing process when the provider obtained a consent for treatment.

Documentation of care coordination activities

Care coordination is a discrete activity that needs to be documented in the chart. This is especially important when the provider needs to document outcomes for individual clients or a particular subset of clients. If care coordination is the major activity performed in the program, the documentation can also be used to support billing, and document that the requirements for a particular grant are being met. The following care coordination activities should always be documented for CYSHN:

- The name of the child's primary care provider (PCP). If the child does not have a PCP, efforts to assist the family to obtain a source of primary care should be documented.

- A list of specialty and community providers, and documentation of any contacts with them.

- Family's financial situation has been assessed – income, insurance, transportation.

- Family's coping skills, strengths, and needs have been documented.

- Documentation has been obtained of referrals made to other providers and the outcome of referrals. Copies of screening results, growth charts, and referral forms are present in chart.

- Documentation has been done of teaching that facilitated a parent or child's coping, self-care, or advocacy skills. This may include teaching a direct skill such as how to do a tube feeding; or if may include teaching communication skills, such as teaching a young teen parent how to communicate with her child's providers in a manner that will result in a positive outcome.

- Evidence was obtained that the care plan was developed in partnership with the family.

- Documentation was obtained of activities related to assisting a teenager to transition to adulthood, if applicable. This activity should be included in all records for children who are 14 years or older.

Finally, the chart can be viewed as chapters in a book. Each chapter is being written about an episode of care, or a period of time in which a provider was working with a child. Each chapter needs to build on the previous chapter. Each note needs to include the provider's assessment of the child's current status, as well as a statement of how well the planned interventions are working. If the interventions are successful, the plan of care should state that the interventions were successful and should continue until the goal is met. If unsuccessful, the plan should document why the intervention was not successful as well as needed changes in the plan (K.K. Farrimond, personal interview, August 22, 2011).

ASSESSMENT, AND DEVELOPMENT
OF AN INTERPROFESSIONAL PLAN
OF CARE

The chart should not be merely a repository of narrative notes and checklists. The lives of cyshn and their families are very complex. Like all families, they experience many episodes of joy and sorrow and as they develop a trusting relationship, the provider will have the privilege of sharing in many of these moments. The chart needs to reflect what life was like for the child and their family and how the provider's interventions made a difference.

A note about electronic health records (EHRS)

In 2009, the federal government passed the American Recovery and Reinvestment Act (ARRA). The part of the act relating to EHRS provides a requirement that healthcare providers adopt electronic health records by 2014, and provides financial incentives for business that adopt EHRS. Initially, this act was passed to facilitate more efficient payment of Medicare and Medicaid claims. As stated in the Federal Register (2010), the intent of the ARRA is to:

> promote the adoption and meaningful use of interoperable health information technology (HIT) and qualified electronic health records (EHRs). These provisions, together with Title XIII of Division A of ARRA, may be cited as the "Health Information Technology for Economic and Clinical Health Act" or the "HITECH Act." These incentive payments are part of a broader effort under the HITECH Act to accelerate the adoption of HIT and utilization of qualified EHRs.

Many health systems and community providers have already adopted EHRS or are in the process of doing so. The process of converting from paper charts to an EHR can be daunting and stressful. However, there are some steps that nurses can take to make the process easier. First of all, nurses should take the time to learn all the intricacies of the record system and develop the skill to chart quickly and accurately. Initially, it will take longer to chart in an EHR than a paper chart. Accurate keyboarding skills are necessary. Nurses must be strong advocates for the needs of their practice and must be an active participant in choosing the criteria for adoption of an EHR by their employer. Large hospital systems frequently have nurse informaticists who can ensure that nursing needs are met. In a community agency, the decision about which system to purchase may have been made by a business manager who did not have an awareness that a system that works well for clinical practice may not work at all for a public health nurse who is doing home visiting. Databases must be customizable to include templates for completing screening forms. The system must be able to record the data that is needed to document grant requirements. It is important to have basic reporting functions built in that can be accessed by staff nurses and managers to monitor the nurse's own practice. Large employers have data analysts on staff who can run more complex reports but community agencies generally do not have this capacity, unless they are a large urban health department.

ASSESSMENT, AND DEVELOPMENT
OF AN INTERPROFESSIONAL PLAN
OF CARE

OTHER RECOMMENDED RESOURCES

Care Coordination within the Medical Home

- **Care Coordination Toolkit from the Center for Children with Special Needs**
  Developed for professionals who coordinate care for children in Washington State. Includes resources for professionals, for families, and for teens and their families. This kit includes resources developed with funding from the Children with Special Health Care Needs (CSHCN) Program of the Washington State Department of Health: http://cshcn.org/professionals

- **Washington Medical Home Leadership Network**

  - Care Coordination within a Medical Home: http://www.medicalhome.org/4Download/carecoord_sep2007.pdf

  - Action Care Plan: http://www.medicalhome.org/4Download/actioncare plan.doc

  - Care Plan for a Child with Special Needs in Child Care:

  Oregon Kids: Healthy and Safe

  Child care health and safety manual – see section on caring for children with special needs https://public.health.oregon.gov/HEALTHYPEOPLEFAMILIES /BABIES/HEALTHCHILDCARE/Pages/okhs.aspx

  Tools to Assess the Complexity of Child and Family Needs

- CaCoon Program Care Coordination Tier Level Assessment: http://www.ohsu.edu/xd/outreach/occyshn/training-education/upload/Tier-Level-Assessment-PHN-Guide.pdf

REFERENCES

Austin, S. (2006). Ladies and gentleman of the jury, I present the nursing documentation. *Nursing 2006, 36*(1), 56–64.

Burns, C.E., & Kodadek, S. (2009). *Child and family health assessment in pediatric primary care*. C.E. Burns, A.M. Dunn, M.A. Brady, et al. (Eds.), Philadelphia, PA: Saunders Elsevier.

CaCoon Health Notes. (May 2011). Retrieved from http://www.ohsu.edu/xd/outreach/occyshn/programs-projects/upload/CaCoon_HealthNotes_2011_MAY .pdf

ASSESSMENT, AND DEVELOPMENT OF AN INTERPROFESSIONAL PLAN OF CARE

CaCoon Program Manual. (2012). Oregon Center for Children and Youth with Special Health Needs, Oregon Health and Science University. For information, contact OCCYSHN at 1–877–307–7070. Web Site: http://www.ohsu.edu/xd/out reach/occyshn/

Child and Adolescent Health Measurement Initiative (CAHMI) (2012). Demographics and CSHCN prevalence for all children ages 0–17. Retrieved from www.cahmi.org

Federal Register. (2010). Health information technology: Initial set of standards, implementation specifications, and certification criteria for electronic health record technology. *Federal Register, 75*(8), January 13, 2010. Washington, DC: US Office of the National Coordinator for Health Information.

Genetic Alliance. (2012). Retrieved from http://www.geneticalliance.org/about

Hoffman, N.A. (2011). The requirements for culturally and linguistically appropriate services in health care. *Journal of Nursing Law, 14*(2), 49–57.

Jack, S.M, DiCenso, A., & Lohfeld, L. (2005). A theory of maternal engagement with public health nurses and family visitors. *Journal of Advanced Nursing, 49,* 182–190.

Lipkin, P.H. (2011). Developmental and behavioral surveillance and screening within the medical home. In R.G. Voight, M.M. Macias, & S.M. Myers (Eds.), *Developmental and Behavioral Pediatrics.* Elk Grove Village, IL: American Academy of Pediatrics.

Lipson, J.G., & Dibble, S.L. (2005) Providing culturally appropriate health care. In J.G. Lipson & S.L. Dibble (Eds.), *Culture and clinical care.* San Francisco, CA: USCF Nursing Press.

Lucas, B.L., Feucht, S.A. Feucht, & Lynn, E. (2004). *Children with special health care needs: Nutrition care handbook.* Pediatric Nutrition Practice Group and Dietetics in Developmental and Psychiatric Disorders. Chicago, IL: American Dietetic Association.

Narramore, N. (2008). Meeting the emotional needs of parents who have a child with complex needs. *Journal of Children's and Young People's Nursing, 2*(3), 103–107.

Smith, K., & Bazini-Barakat, N. (2003). A public health nursing practice model: Melding public health principles with the nursing process. *Public Health Nursing, 20*(1), 42–48.

OTHER RECOMMENDED READINGS

Barnett, D., Clements, M., Kaplan-Estrin, M., & Fialka, J. (2003). Building new dreams: Supporting parents' adaptation to their child with special needs. *Infants and Young Children, 16,* 184–200.

Cervasio, K. (2010). The role of the pediatric home health care nurse. *Home Health Care Nurse, 28*(7) 424–431.

Gordon, J.B., Colby, H.H., Bartelt, T., et al. (2007). A tertiary care-primary care partnership model for medically complex and fragile children and youth with special health care needs *Archives of Pediatric Adolescent Medicine 16*(10), 937–944.

Josten, L.V.E., Savik, K., Anderson, M.R., et al. (2002). Dropping out of maternal and child home visits. *Public Health Nursing, 19,* 3–10. doi: 10.1046/j.1525-1446.2002.d19002.x

Lundberg, C., Warren, J., Brokel, J., et al. (2008). Selecting a standardized ter-

ASSESSMENT, AND DEVELOPMENT OF AN INTERPROFESSIONAL PLAN OF CARE

minology for the electronic health record that reveals the impact of nursing on patient care. *Online Journal of Nursing Informatics (OJNI)*, *12*, (2). Available at http:ojni.org/12_2/lundberg.pdf

Robinson, K.M. (2010.) Care coordination: A priority for health reform. *Policy Politics Nursing Practice*, *11*, 266–274.

Young, K.T., Davis, K., Schoen, C., & Parker, S.(1998). Listening to parents: A national survey of parents with young children. *Archives of Pediatric Adolescent Medicine 152*(3), 255–262.

ASSESSMENT, AND DEVELOPMENT
OF AN INTERPROFESSIONAL PLAN
OF CARE

Caring for Children with Special Healthcare Needs and Their Families: A Handbook for Healthcare Professionals, First Edition. Edited by Linda L. Eddy.
© 2013 John Wiley & Sons, Inc. Published 2013 by John Wiley & Sons, Inc.

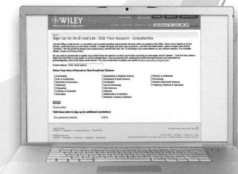